STOP DIETING
and START
LOSING WEIGHT

JEN BREWER, RD

STOP
DIETING
and START
LOSING WEIGHT

JEN BREWER, RD

Plain Sight Publishing
An Imprint of Cedar Fort, Inc.
Springville, Utah

ISBN 13: 978-1-4621-1063-6

Published by Plain Sight Publishing, an imprint of Cedar Fort, Inc.
2373 W. 700 S., Springville, UT 84663
Distributed by Cedar Fort, Inc. www.cedarfort.com

LIBRARY OF CONGRESS CATALOGING-IN-PUBLICATION DATA

Brewer, Jen, 1974- , author.
 Stop dieting and start losing weight : 25 lifestyle changes to control your weight for good / Jen Brewer, RD.
     pages cm
 Includes bibliographical references and index.
 ISBN 978-1-4621-1063-6 (alk. paper)
 1. Weight loss. I. Title.

 RM222.2.B757 2012
 613.2'5--dc23
                                                    2012034825

Cover design by Erica Dixon
Cover design © 2012 by Lyle Mortimer
Edited and typeset by Emily S. Chambers

Printed in the United States of America

10 9 8 7 6 5 4 3 2 1

This book is dedicated to:

My Mom: Whom I still call for help in the kitchen.

My Dad: Who stayed up way too late way too many nights helping me hone countless writing assignments throughout my schooling years.

My Husband: Who helped encourage me to write by telling his colleagues, patients, and everyone he knows that I "had a book coming out"—before one word was ever put to paper.

My Children: Who inspire me everyday . . . and provide brutally honest opinions on my cooking endeavors—the good, the bad, and the downright inedible.

Contents

Acknowledgments 1

Section 1: The Diet Dilemma 3

The Problem with Diets 5

Your Lifetime Eating Program 8

Motivation 10

How to Use This Book 12

Section 2: Principles of Weight Management . . 15

  1. Calorie Output Should Exceed Input. 16

  2. Balance Your Basic Body Ingredients. 19

  3. Get Enough Sleep 26

  4. Exercise 27

Section 3: Tools 31

  1. Pay Cash for Your Calories. 32

  2. Slendersize 34

  3. Eat by Volume 36

  4. Subtract by Addition 39

  5. Relax and Enjoy. 41

  6. Eat Offensively, Not Defensively 42

  7. Eat Close to the Farm 44

  8. Use the Apple Test 45

  9. Drink Lots of Water. 46

 10. Keep a Food Journal 48

 11. Use a Food-Group Checklist 49

 12. Eat Mindfully 50

 13. Face Your Stuff, Don't Stuff Your Face. . . . 52

14. Eat Breakfast 54
15. Take Control of the Restaurant Scene 56
16. Shop Deliberately. 59
17. Plan Menus 61
18. Eat to End Hunger, Not to Feel Full 62
19. Stop the Stress 63
20. Schedule Exercise. 68
21. Don't Be a Garbage Disposal 73
22. Look Long, Step Small 75
23. Use the Buddy System 77
24. Weigh In Weekly. 78
25. Use Meal Replacements 79

Section 4: What's in Your Toolbox? 81

Appendices 103

Appendix A: Carbohydrates. 103
Appendix B: Protein 106
Appendix C: Fats 107
Appendix D: Vitamins and Minerals 108
Appendix E: Basal Metabolic Rate. 119
Appendix F: Calorie Dollars 120
Appendix G: Food Diary Example. 121
Appendix H: Food Group Checklists. 122
Appendix I: Stop Sign 129
Appendix J: Recipes 130
Appendix K: Meal-Planning Worksheet. 135

References 137

About the Author. 159

Acknowledgments

This book exists today because of the work of incredibly talented people. Emily Chambers's final editing took the book to a whole new level. David Cheney's artistic talent made the pictures inside take on a life of their own. The team at Cedar Fort took my original book, waved their magic wands, and made it even better than I could imagine.

And, finally, I hold a huge debt of gratitude for the bookends of my formal education: Susan Smith, my first grade teacher, who taught me that if I chewed my carrots last at lunch, they would help "brush my teeth"—opening my eyes to the wonder of food. And Dr. Nora Nyland, as well as the entire incredible dietetics education staff at BYU, who taught me a whole lot about nutrition, and even more about life.

Thank you.

THE DIET DILEMMA

If you're trying to lose weight, or even live healthier, there is no shortage of advice. Month after month, almost every magazine in the checkout line touts "The new miracle diet" or the "breakthrough pill that will end your dieting woes!" I especially love the ones that say "Lose 20 Pounds by Christmas"—in the December issue. In fact, google the word diet and you will be hit with over 330 million responses in 0.15 seconds. Good luck with that. Let's face it: if you drop the calorie intake enough, any diet will work to take pounds off. If you stick with it. Forever.

"Of course you lost weight on the cabbage diet; you got so bored eating only cabbage that you just stopped eating altogether! "
—Jay Leno

The Problem with Diets

❝ I've been on a constant diet for the last two decades. I've lost a total of 789 pounds. By all accounts, I should be hanging from a charm bracelet.❞

—Erma Bombeck

The traditional use of the word *diet* has changed over the years. Originally the definition of *diet* was "what a person or animal usually eats and drinks; daily fare"[1] (as in, the Viking diet consisted of . . .). It referred to what a person ate consistently throughout his or her lifespan.

The word has evolved to mean a temporary change in eating habits. Our language reflects this change in word meaning: "I'm going on a diet." Although no one says it out loud, the rest of the sentence is implied: ". . . so at some point, I will be going off a diet."

Fad diets are powerful in our culture because they are started by companies that are after profits—not pounds. They have *one* goal: to make money. They often enlist false testimonials with paid actors claiming to have lost vast amounts of weight. As the novelty of a fad wears off, marketers start promoting a new one.

Be especially wary of any diet that requires you to buy (and keep on buying) the powder, pill, potion, or packet. It will not work for you in the long run.

I could fill this whole book dissecting specific diets, but I won't because:

1. That would take the rest of the book.

2. By the time this book hits the press, the list would already be obsolete, since more and more diets hit the stands daily.

Chances are, the celery-and-peanut-butter diet that helped your neighbor lose 50 pounds would be horrible for you. And in fact it will be horrible for your neighbor if he cannot stay on the program long-term. There is no "one size fits all" approach to a healthy lifestyle.

Here is an overly simplified yet too true synopsis of the cycle of fad diets: Years ago fat was declared as the "bad guy," and people bought into it. They changed what they ate. Since lowfat and fat-free products weren't readily available, they changed what they ate—oftentimes cooking at home from scratch (gasp!) and experimenting with new, healthier foods.

Food production companies also bought into it and started producing "lowfat," "light," and "fat-free" versions of some of our favorite foods. Once people started seeing their favorites in the stores with the new and improved labels with less fat (although not altering the bottom line: calories), people reverted back to eating their "normal" fare—and more often than not, eating more than they had before (it's fat-free, so I can eat twice as much!). Waistlines continued to expand.

Enter carbohydrates into the "bad guy" role. Once

again, people bought into it. They changed what they ate, again starting to cook from home and experiment with different foods. Food production companies also jumped on board (are you seeing a trend here?), and our favorite foods in "low carbohydrate" versions started appearing on store shelves once again. Eating reverted back, and so did waistlines.

Next on the cycle came gluten. Do I even need to repeat the explanation again? I remember walking into the store to see a "gluten free" cookie. And I knew the cycle was about to come full force once again.

Despite this overabundance of "solutions," the obesity rate has continued to grow. From 1990 to 2006, the average obesity rate skyrocketed from under 15 percent of the population in most states to over 20 percent in all states. That means one in every five people is obese. Two states even reported obesity rates of over 30 percent. That's one out of every three people! In the three subsequent years, eight more states went over 30 percent. Epidemic? Absolutely.[2–6]

Obesity consumes vast amounts of time, energy, and resources and leaves immeasurable personal devastation in its wake. In February 2010, the Center for Disease Control (CDC) estimated direct and indirect health costs due to obesity at $147 billion. In 2006, each obese patient spent an average of $1,429 more on health care than his or her regular-weight counterparts.[7] Many diseases have been shown to be directly or indirectly linked to obesity, including heart disease, diabetes, hypertension, hypercholesterolemia, stroke, respiratory diseases (sleep apnea, asthma), osteoarthritis, gynecological and pregnancy complications, and cancer—just to name a few.[8,9]

Obesity also has psychosocial implications. Although larger body sizes have been associated with affluence throughout history, in our modern society, having a body mass index in the obese range leads to social stigmas. Obesity also has been shown to have some link to fewer years of education, lower levels of income, and lower rates of marriage.[10]

> **"**I have gained and lost the same ten pounds so many times over and over again, my cellulite must have déjà vu.**"**
>
> —Jane Wagner

The bottom line: it doesn't matter who we label as the "bad guy," if we don't change what we eat and how we live, we will never see a change in our waistlines and our weight lines.

Your Lifetime Eating Program

My advice: stop dieting. Start eating. Start eating in a way that helps your body become the healthy, strong body you want. Create your own personalized eating program. You can include in this program the foods that you love (in moderation). The only way to control your weight for the rest of your life is to get on an eating program for the rest of your life. If you love triple-fudge chocolate cake, then include that in your eating program—just not every day. The best way to know if an eating program will work for you is to ask yourself, "How long can I do this?" As much as we crave a quick and easy fix, permanent weight control can only be achieved with a permanent change in nutrition and behavior.

Research backs this up. A study performed by Harvard physicians followed people for two years on various diets—all focused on different nutrients (high-fat, low-fat, high-protein, low-carbohydrate, and so on), but with similar overall calories. At the end of two years, people in every group who completed the program (those who stuck with it and didn't give up) lost weight.[11] Yes, any sound diet works. If you stay with it. Forever.

With the right eating program, after a slip, a binge, or vacation eating, you can resume the program quickly, without a lot of damage, emotional pressure, or negative self-talk. This individualized program will likely only produce a weekly weight loss of one or two pounds. However, the goal is not to drop weight quickly—the goal is to maintain the weight loss for years to come.

Unfortunately with yo-yo dieting (going on and off diets), after the diet is discarded, the weight comes back quickly. Often the dieter gains back even more weight and becomes heavier then before the diet began.[12–14] Some research has even shown that yo-yo dieting can also impair the immune system, cause slightly elevated blood pressure, and lower the levels of HDL (the good cholesterol).[15]

If you can find an eating program that you can maintain indefinitely, you can manage your weight effectively—for the rest of your life. That is the point of this book—to help you find an eating program that works for you.

No doubt you have talked to friends and relatives who have found their miracle weight-loss program and think it will work for everyone. This book will not give the magic pill to the wonderful world of weight loss. This book is meant to be used as your personal nutrition toolbox to create your lifelong plan to a healthier you. Not your uncle's or neighbor's or friend's plan—your plan.

Motivation

" In order to change, we must be sick and tired of being sick and tired.**"**

—*Author Unknown*

Motivation to build a healthy body is twofold. First, you must come to a point at which your desire to change outweighs your desire to remain heavy and unhealthy. All of the information in the world is not going to do you a bit of good if you are not ready to change.

Take a moment and really ask yourself, what is driving you to become healthier? A doctor's visit? Your tight-fitting clothes? An upcoming high school reunion? A wedding? Whatever the reason, your motivation to achieve lifelong, sustainable change must be stronger than your desire for overeating here and now.

Change is hard. There is no getting around it. The second step of motivation to build a healthy life will keep you going, even when you step on the scale (after working like crazy to overcome your old habits) and learn that you have only lost one measly pound, or nothing at all. The body changes will come, but they won't come overnight. This part of motivation surfaces after the big "New Year's Party" has ended. Every moment of every day, the desire to keep working on a healthier you must be more important than the desire to quit. This is what keeps you on track when you are constantly bombarded with the temptation to put trash into your body. It's this type of motivation that overrides the three o'clock in the afternoon, gotta-have-chocolate-or-die feeling.

Your decision to embark on a healthier lifestyle will not be a tiptoe-through-the-tulips kind of a change. You need to just accept that fact and be ready for the obstacles. They will come. When they come, you have two choices: you can either view each obstacle as a wall to stop your progress, or you turn them into stepping-stones to reach new heights. You have the power to decide which way it will be.

This requires a new way of thinking about food and eating. You must find yourself looking for ways to stay on the healthy path instead of looking for excuses to fall off. The excuses and self-doubt will always be in the back of your mind. You can acknowledge those thoughts but not give in to them. Let them come, and then let them leave. They do not define you. You choose how to define you.

Simply learning more will not motivate you. Somewhere along the way, you must put into practice what you are learning. Start today. Pick one tool. Any tool. Pick the one that speaks to you the loudest. Implement it now. Turn it into a habit. Then move on to the next tool.

You will stumble. You will fall. The key is to get up and keep moving forward every time that happens. It's not in the falling that you fail—it's in the failing to get back up. Every time you get back on track, you are that much closer to your goal.

How to Use This Book

Who has time to sit down and read a book from cover to cover (unless it's about a wizard or a vampire)? This book is a reference tool. If you scan the table of contents, you will find that some of the subjects naturally speak to you. Start there. Heck, start at the last chapter if you want. Each chapter is a tool that can help you start building a healthier, sustainable eating pattern. Find what works for you; ignore the rest. (I won't be offended, I promise!)

Here's a good rule of thumb to follow with this book: when you read something and say to yourself, "Hey, that sounds feasible. I could do that," then that is something that is going to work for you. Circle, underline, or just rip it out (one usable page is a thousand times better then an entire unread book). Put it in your personal arsenal of "healthy living helps" to get you on your road to a better body and a healthier life.

The remainder of this book is divided into three sections: Principles, Tools, and What's in Your Toolbox (personal stories).

Principles are the overarching and unchanging standards. They pass the test of time, science, and research as to how to live the healthiest life. They don't change, and we can't cheat them and get away with it in the long run.

Tools are a collection of techniques to implement these principles. When a carpenter decides to build a house, he doesn't just grab a hammer and use only it from beginning to end. He needs several different tools for different steps, challenges, and situations in order to build the most stable, beautiful structure.

The tools that we use to build our personal eating plans will be very specific and different for each individual. For example, green spinach smoothies for breakfast may work great for one person but make the next person feel deprived and bitter.

If a nutrition program makes you feel deprived and bitter, you will not stay on it long term. Different situations, different people—even different days—require different tools to achieve an optimally healthy body.

Finally, the What's in Your Toolbox? section included in this book shows you how real people have used the Principles and Tools from this book (or forged their own personal tools) to lose weight and keep it off.

PRINCIPLES OF WEIGHT MANAGEMENT

Fads fade. Principles are forever. The four tried-and-true principles in this section will help you understand how to keep your body healthy and manage your weight. There are many ways to go about following the principles, but the principles will never change.

Principle 1: Calorie Output Should Exceed Input

This is the basic law of weight management: if you take in (eat) more than you work off (through exercise, your basal metabolism, and so on), you will gain weight. If you take in less than you work off, you will lose weight. This can be accomplished in three ways:

1. Eat less (fewer calories).

2. Exercise more.

3. Eat less and exercise more.

The healthiest way to lose weight is to lose at a rate of one to two pounds per week. One pound of fat is equal to 3,500 calories. So if you want to lose one pound of body weight in one week, you will have to find a way to create a 3,500-calorie deficit in your body. If you want to lose two pounds in a week, you will need to create a 7,000-calorie deficit. That breaks down to 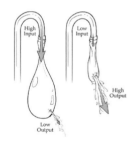 500 or 1,000 calories a day, respectively, that you need to shave off of your intake, or work off with exercise.

Every body uses a certain amount of calories each day just to survive. This is called your basal metabolic rate (BMR). Some sources also use the term resting metabolic rate (RMR). There are many different theories and ways to estimate your own basal metabolic rate (see Appendix E to figure out yours). Many factors beyond basic survival will increase the amount of calories your body uses (exercise, working, sickness, and so on).

To figure out the net number of calories your body requires to meet your weight-management goals, just do the math: calculate your basal metabolic rate, adjust it for your activity level (see Appendix E), then subtract the number of calories that correspond with your weight-loss goals (for example, subtract 500 calories a day to lose a pound a week). This number becomes your daily caloric goal. When you want to eat more, add enough exercise to offset the extra calories.

Many people try to overcomplicate the simple input/output rule, either to make excuses for why they can't shed the pounds or to sell a particular diet plan. Here are a couple of common myths:

Myth #1: It's all in the genes.

I have heard this excuse almost more than any other: "I just don't have the right genes." "Why does so-and-so get to eat all she wants and never gain a pound, when I gain five pounds just by looking at food?" Or, "My parents have 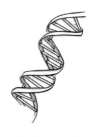 always been big; there's just nothing I can do about it."

Yes, some people have been blessed with great genes

(and also blessed to fit into great jeans). Though it may not look like it on the outside, their bodies are still working off more calories due to their high metabolism, and, therefore, they can eat more and still look great (dang it!).

Genetics plays a role in our metabolism, and our upbringing does too—some of our food preferences have to do with what we were served by Mom and Dad in our early years. Genetics also plays a role in our risk for certain diseases.

You have two choices when it comes to genetics. You can let it overtake you and put you in the victim seat, or you can take the bull by the horns and change what you have the power to change within your genetic parameters.

When we start working within our own means and not stressing about our genes, we realize how much control we really do have over our lives and our health.

Myth #2: Calories count more at night.

Late-night eating has become taboo in the dieting world. Some diets tout an eating plan that has you stop eating at 6:00 p.m. (or any random time). Here's the fact—your body does 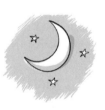 not have an alarm clock that suddenly sounds at 6:00 p.m. and states, "I have now passed the calorie-burning phase and will begin the calorie-storing phase, so anything you eat after this point turns into fat." Yes, this sounds absurd, but that's essentially what that diet plan is trying to feed you—after you have paid up, of course.

The real underlying problem with eating at night is that by the time you have eaten throughout the day and finished dinner, you are most likely at your calorie limit, if not over it. When you sit down to watch TV and grab a snack, you are overloading your body's calorie level and those extra calories get stored as fat—due to the amount of food that you have already eaten throughout the day, not the specific time at which you are now eating.

The other problem is that at night while you're watching TV, you don't normally reach for carrots and Brussels sprouts—you typically go for chips, ice cream, cookies, and other foods that tend to be higher in fat and calories and lower in nutritional quality, which again leads to an overload of calories.[16–20]

Principle 2: Balance Your Basic Body Ingredients

So it's really all about calories, right? Well, yes and no. Calories count, but the type of calories you eat also matter. This principle was illustrated in a conversation with my amazing, junk-food-loving brother:

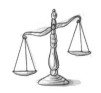

"If it's all about the calories, can I just determine how many calories I need, and then eat my calorie load in donuts and cheeseburgers? As long as I stay under my calorie limit, I'll still lose weight, right?"

On one hand, that's true, a person will lose weight by staying in calorie-withdrawal mode (eating less than the body works off). But there is so much to be said about the value of the calories that go into the body. The human body cannot function on calories alone. It requires many different nutrients. If you cut off all but those that come from donuts and cheeseburgers, you will actually do significant harm to your body in the long run.

> "More die in the United States of too much food than of too little."
> —John Kenneth Galbraith, *The Affluent Society*

This is the underlying cause of a new phenomenon spreading throughout our nation: too many people are overweight and undernourished. They have gotten an overabundance of calories from the wrong sources and therefore have gotten bigger while starving their bodies of what they really need to function effectively. We are literally eating ourselves to death.

Our bodies need six ingredient categories every day, in varying quantities, in order to function efficiently:

1. Carbohydrates
2. Protein
3. Fat

] MACRO

4. Vitamins
5. Minerals
6. Water

] micronutrients

The three macronutrients (carbohydrates, protein, and fat) actually supply calories for the body. The three micronutrients (vitamins, minerals, water) don't supply calories; they supply various nutrients that are vital for optimal health.

Carbohydrates

Carbohydrates are the fuel for the body. If you don't put gas in your car, it won't run for long. If you don't replenish your carbohydrate stores, your body won't run efficiently for long.

In fact, the only form of energy that the brain can use is glucose—the broken-down form of carbohydrates. If you starve your body of carbohydrates, your body will make glucose from other sources, but in the process it also produces waste products that have to go to the liver to be detoxified, and then to the kidneys to be flushed out. Maintaining such a pattern year in and year out could eventually overload both the liver and kidneys. Not exactly optimal living.

The current recommendations for carbohydrate intake vary, but generally, between 45 to 65 percent of calories should come from carbohydrates, preferably from whole grain or complex sources (see Appendix A for more information on carbohydrates). [21–22]

If carbohydrates are so important for the body, why do they get such a bad rap? It's a matter of the type and amount of carbohydrate that we put into our bodies.

There are basically two main types of carbohydrates:

simple and complex. Simple carbohydrates are just that, simple sugars. The body doesn't have to work very hard to get the energy from this source, and therefore it is pretty easy to overeat these types of carbohydrates and have the body kick it into storage, which increases fat stores and potentially leads to weight gain and obesity. Simple sugars are found mostly in refined foods (white sugar, packaged snack foods, and so on).

Complex carbohydrates are, well, a bit more structurally complex. These carbohydrates make the body work just to digest them, therefore burning more calories even in the digestion process. Complex carbohydrates also have many added benefits and include other nutrients.

One of the most important subcategories of complex carbohydrates is fiber. Ahh, yes, fiber! This is a hot topic in our culture, and there is good reason for that. Fiber plays a huge role in our overall health. Fiber has been proven to benefit the body in many ways, most notably its role in lowering cholesterol and decreasing the risk for certain types of cancer. There are two types of fiber, as illustrated in Appendix A. The recommendations are to consume between 25 grams (for women) and 38 grams (for men) of fiber each day. For Americans, the average intake of fiber is 12 to 15 grams—not even half of the upper recommendation![23–24]

To identify complex carbohydrates, think brown— brown rice, wheat bread, bran cereal, and so on. Fruits and vegetables are also great sources of fiber, especially the peelings, which are generally full of fiber. Did you know you can even eat the peel of a kiwi? (Not the most

palatable way to get your fiber, but doable, nonetheless.)
See Tool 4: Subtract by Addition and Appendix A for
ways to increase fiber intake.

Protein

Protein breaks down into building blocks for
the body. Think of a box of Legos. You can build any
number of structures from all of the different types of
pieces. This is like protein. When you eat protein, your
body breaks it down into tiny pieces called amino acids.

The body requires over 20 types of amino acids.
Once it has all of these tiny pieces, it can then go to
work building different components, such as immuno-
proteins, enzymes, and hormones.

Protein also helps the body by providing structure,
helping to build cells and muscles, enabling fetal growth,
repairing wounds, and aiding the immune system. Nine
of the 20 amino acids are called essential amino acids—
the body cannot produce them; they have to be eaten in
different types of protein rich foods.[23]

Many people think that eating protein will auto-
matically make you bulky and muscle-bound, but the
intake of protein is only one side of the equation—you
must work the muscles to be able to put the protein to
work and help muscles grow.

The current recommendation for protein intake, by
some sources, is to eat about 0.8 grams of protein for
each kilogram of body weight.[25] Roughly translated, a
150-pound woman should take in 54 grams of protein a

day. Other sources recommend an average intake of 46 grams per day for women and 71 grams for men.[26]

Complete protein foods (those that have all of the essential amino acids) are meats, eggs, and dairy. Complementary foods each have some essential amino acids and can be paired together to provide complete protein. These pairings include beans and rice (or tortillas), peas and toast, pasta and cheese, peanut butter and bread, and hummus and pita bread. (See Appendix B for more information on protein.)

Fat

Yes, the body needs fat. It just doesn't need very much of it. Fat has many functions in the body. It provides cushion for the organs and bones, it transports some of the vitamins (vitamins A, D, E, and K), and it provides insulation for the body.[23]

Many food groups give the body ample amounts of fat. It's one thing that you do not have to search for each day. Don't worry, it will find you. The recommendation is to keep fat calories below 20 to 35 percent of the overall intake of calories (no more than 10 percent from saturated fat).[23]

There are three main types of fat: saturated, monounsaturated, and polyunsaturated. The saturation level mainly describes the bonding of hydrogen in the fat molecule. In saturated fat, every available carbon-hydrogen bond is attached to a hydrogen molecule. In monounsaturated fat, there is one double bond. In polyunsaturated fats, two or more bonds are double bonds. (See Appendix C for pictures of fat molecules).

The worst form of fat for the body is saturated fat. This is the type of fat that leads to atherosclerosis (hardening of the arteries) and increased cholesterol levels. Trans fat is a man-made fat through the process of hydrogenation to provide a more structurally stable fat molecule (this helps with shelf life, but not with health!). Although it is more stable in food, trans fat is no better than saturated fat in its effects on human health.[27–29]

Monounsaturated and polyunsaturated fat, although they provide a lot of calories for the body, don't directly increase cholesterol levels.

Vitamins and Minerals

The body needs a whole slew of vitamins and minerals to function efficiently. Vitamins and minerals don't supply direct energy (calories) to the body; they act as catalysts for many functions of the body and are vital to survival.

Vitamins and minerals are organic compounds found naturally in foods (and sometimes the soil in which the food is grown). Most vitamins and minerals can't be synthesized by the body and, most important, cause a specific deficiency syndrome when they are absent from the body.

See Appendix D for a list of common vitamins and minerals and their functions.

Water

The function of water is simple: if you don't have it, you die. It makes up 60 to 80 percent of body weight.

Pretty much everything that happens in the body requires the use of water. It aids in body temperature regulation, digestion, metabolism, and nutrient transport, just to name a few.

The current recommendation for water intake is at least 8 to 10 cups of water every day. (See Tool 9: Drink Lots of Water for tips on how to increase your water intake).

Principle 3: Get Enough Sleep

Sleep is one of the lesser-known principles for weight control. Simply put: get enough sleep. It helps the body and mind regroup, but, more important, it helps all of the body systems run more efficiently, including metabolism.

In our culture, people use their lack of sleep almost as a bragging right as they talk about who needs the least amount of sleep. What they don't realize is that lack of sleep sabotages weight loss.

Studies on sleep show that many hormones become imbalanced if the body is not allowed the right amount of sleep (for most people that figure is seven to nine hours a night). Ghrelin, 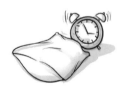 the hormone that causes hunger, actually increases in sleep-deprived individuals, and leptin, the hormone that tells your brain it's time to stop eating, decreases.[30-44]

What's more, when people are tired, they are less

likely to hit the gym and more likely to grab a quick snack or cup of coffee to stay awake or to slump on the couch, reaching for comfort foods.[41]

Principle 4: Exercise

Our bodies were created to work. In our society, we are constantly looking for ways to get around this simple principle of work. We have convenienced and automated ourselves into obesity.

The principle of exercise is basic: you've got to move it to lose it.

Here is a simple scenario: as discussed in Principle 1, it takes a deficit of 3,500 calories to lose one pound. To reach that goal in a week, you would need to cut back on 500 calories every day. To lose two pounds, you'd have to cut 1,000 calories every day. That's a lot of calories to cut.

However, if you add exercise, you can alter the amount of calories you need to cut, or, even better, you might not

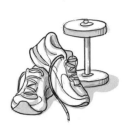

have to cut any calories at all. Sixty minutes of walking (at 3.5 mph) for a 200-pound person burns 346 calories, so if you did this activity six days a week, you would burn 2,422 calories. That would allow you to meet your goal of losing one pound

a week with a cutback of only 154 calories a day. If you want to go for two pounds, you'd have to cut your calories by 654 per day.[45] That's a big difference, just by adding exercise.

There are two main types of exercise: aerobic (also called cardio) and anaerobic (sometimes called resistance training). Aerobic exercise is anything that is continuous in nature and consists of moving the same muscle groups for a prolonged period of time (at least 10 minutes). Examples of aerobic exercise include walking, jogging, swimming, and biking.

Anaerobic exercise (resistance or strength training) uses the muscles to work against a resistive load (usually weights, bands, medicine balls, and so on).

The body needs both forms of exercise throughout the week. The current recommendations say that we should aim for at least 60 minutes of exercise every day of the week. Of those bouts of exercise, two to three sessions should be resistance training (preferably alternating the days with cardio), and the rest should be aerobic activity. With resistance training, it's best to lift muscle groups that oppose each other in the same session. For example, biceps (front of upper arms) and triceps (back of upper arms), pectoralis (chest) and trapezius (upper back), deltoids (shoulders) and latissimus dorsi (lats) (middle back), abductors and adductors (inner and outer thighs), and quadriceps (front of leg), and hamstrings (back of leg).

One of the biggest complaints I receive from patients regarding exercise is, "I don't have time to exercise." And they are right. We don't have time to exercise. We have to make time to exercise. If you can't find a continuous 60 minutes, you can exercise in smaller sessions throughout the day, provided those sessions increase the heart rate enough to give one the benefits of exercise. In studies, people who exercised for 10-minute mini-sessions throughout the day saw the same benefits as those who did the full amount of exercise at once.[62, 63] See Tool 20: Schedule Exercise for more information on exercise.

Exercise not only aids in weight loss and maintenance but also helps in myriad ways to improve the health of the body.[18,19, 23, 46–61]

I hope this is not completely new information to you. We live in an age where we are absolutely inundated with nutrition information. When I sit down for a consult with a client, rarely do they need me to explain the basics of eating. We all have at least a vague idea of what is healthy for our bodies and what is not. Yet there seems to be a crevice between what we know and what we do. (I was explaining this to a weight loss group once, and one of the sweet ladies jumped right in and was quick to correct me, "No, honey, it's not a crevice, it's a canyon!") So be it a crevice for some, or the grand canyon for others, the point is that what we know doesn't match what we do. How can we overcome that? We need to start small and build a bridge over that gap. The tools that we use and the type of bridge we build are different for everyone, but we need to commit to keep moving to get our actions in harmony with our knowledge. The next section, Tools, will show you just how to do that.

Health Benefits of Exercise

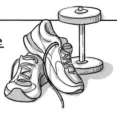

↑ Increases flexibility

↑ Increases strength

↑ Increases blood supply to muscles and organs

↑ Increased HDL cholesterol (the good type of cholesterol

↑ Builds and maintains healthy muscles, bones, and joints

↑ Improves psychological well-being

↑ Enhances work, recreation, and sport performance

↑ Improves glucose tolerance and reduces insulin resistance

↓ Reduces risk of heart disease

↓ Reduces high blood pressure or risk of developing it

↓ Reduces high cholesterol or risk of devoloping it

↓ Reduces risk of developing certain types of cancer

↓ Reduces risk of developing diabetes

↓ Reduces depression and anxiety

↓ Decreases triglycerides

↓ Lowers heart rate

↓ Reduces risk of premature death

• Helps control blood-sugar levels in patients with diabetes

TOOLS

Consider this section your personal toolbox to help you craft healthy nutrition patterns. You don't have to use every tool. Let me repeat that: *you don't have to use every tool.* Just as a carpenter uses a variety of tools to build a mansion, so too should you use a variety of the following tools to create and reshape your personal mansion: your body. Your job in crafting your personal healthy lifestyle is to read through the following chapters and find the few that work for you—the ones that you read and think, "Hey, that makes sense. I could do that!"

Tool 1: Pay Cash for Your Calories

The same principle that got us into the economic crisis in this country also got us into our weight crisis: living on borrowed credit (or on borrowed calories).

Many of us eat more than our allotted calories early each day and then live on a credit system for the

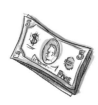

rest of the day (borrowing calories from tomorrow's budget). Much like credit spending, we don't notice all of the little purchases that we make on credit until we get the bill and are blown away by

how much we now owe the creditors. With our body, the little caloric overindulgences go into storage. We don't notice the tiny changes until we get the notice for the high school reunion in the mail and then look in the mirror, horrified.

The little bites do add up—yes, even what Dominique Adair, MS, RD, calls the BLTs (the bites, licks, and tastes) can overdraw our calorie account for the day.

Think of your daily allotment of calories as a bank account. Each day you have an allotted amount of calories to "spend"—your calorie budget. You can determine your budget by calculating your basal metabolic rate (see

Appendix E). This will give you a ballpark figure of the amount of calories your body spends on daily activities, not including exercise.

For example, a five-foot-eight, 35-year-old woman weighing 150 pounds would have a resting BMR of roughly 1,500 calories. If she is lightly active during a normal day, the total calories spent would be 1,850. Moderate activity would increase that figure to 2,100. So each day she can spend between 1,850 and 2,100 calories (depending on activity level) to stay at her current weight.

To remind yourself to stay within your dietary budget, pay cash for your calories. You can track your caloric spending in a variety of ways—charts, balance sheets, Internet tracking programs, phone apps, or mental notes. You can even cut out the "money" in Appendix F (or download from the website all-diets-work.com), count out cash to represent the calories you can spend for the day, and literally carry it with you to pay for the calories as you go.

The key is to be honest and consistent throughout the day (even counting those just-a-little-taste moments). You also need to find a way that works for you to record your calories at the point of purchase, accounting for them in the moment, not in a passive review at the end of the day. Studies have shown that when people try to recall their food intake after the fact, they underestimate what they eat (by as much as 30 percent) and overestimate how much they exercise.[64-79]

The beauty of this system is that you can fit your favorite foods into your budget, you just need to pay for them. Even better, pay ahead. If you know you have a dinner party coming up at your favorite restaurant and you are dying to have the chocolate lava cake, pay for it ahead of time. Set aside the calories for that dish first thing in the morning. Just imagine how much more you will enjoy that cake, knowing you paid cash up front, so you don't have to owe anything to your calorie budget the morning after. You'll be able to stop saying, "Oh man, it's going to take four hours at the gym to burn this thing off!"

My dad taught me an important lesson about this when I was in college. I was at home visiting for the weekend, and we were talking about desserts that we loved. My mom loves cheesecake, and I asked my dad if he loved it too. His reply has come back to me many times, "Oh, I like it okay, but not enough to spend the calories on it—I would rather have something else for that amount of calories."

What wise council: know yourself well enough to know what foods you would rather spend your calories on.

Tool 2: Slendersize

" My doctor told me to stop having intimate dinners for four. Unless there are three other people.**"**

—Orson Wells

We live in a culture of supersizing. When McDonald's first opened its doors in 1955, it only had one hamburger size: 1.6 ounces. Now the largest size is a whopping 8 ounces. French fries started at 2.4 ounces. Now the large weighs in at 6 ounces. Large soft drinks increased from 7 ounces to 32 ounces.[80,81]

Is it any wonder that we have gotten bigger over the years? What we perceive as normal today is actually anywhere from 75 to 500 percent bigger than what was normal not too many years ago. There is no shortage of studies to show that our portion distortion is out of control.[82–88] In fact, in some parts of Europe, the ice cream sizes read: small, medium, large, extra large—and American. It's well known not only in America but also around the globe. Americans like to eat, and we like to eat *big*.

It's time to slendersize. We need to retrain our eyes to size up a true serving. The simplest way to accomplish this is to break out the measuring cups and kitchen scale. No, I'm not kidding (I said it was simple; not easy, fast, or convenient!). Try this: get your normal cereal bowl, pour what you typically eat in the morning, and write down how much you think it is. Now measure how much is actually in it. Surprised?

When I try this in weight-loss classes, the participants are always surprised to see how much restaurant supersizing has affected our everyday eating.

I also ask participants in my classes to use different sizes of plates and bowls to portion out food. Almost across the board, those with bigger plates and bowls pour bigger portions.

The easy answer to this is to downsize your dishes! If you have kids at home, use the toddler-size plates. If you don't have kids at home, go get some smaller plates, bowls, and even utensils.

Here's an example: One serving of ice cream = ½ cup. If you put ½ cup of ice cream in a big ice cream bowl, you will most likely feel a bit deprived. Put that same amount of ice cream in a little parfait cup and suddenly you are having a fancy dessert.

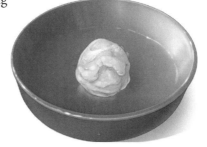

Tool 3: Eat by Volume

If you are the type of person who just likes to eat, then this tool is for you. In fact, whole books have been written on this subject. [89-90] The essence is that by changing what you eat, you can actually eat more food while consuming fewer calories. For a vivid example: think a bowl of chips versus a bowl of salad. Munching on the chips will most likely overload your body with

calories before you feel physically full. On the flip side, you can eat the entire bowl of salad and not come close to overloading on calories (that is, if you skip all of the high-calorie condiments).

Even the same food can be eaten in abundance if it is simply prepared a different way. Take the potato, for example. You could eat 20 (thin) french fries (less than the amount in a Happy Meal!) and get 220 calories, or go for a medium baked potato, getting more food for only 155 calories (without the high-fat condiments).

Different cuts of meat also play by this tool. If you are a meat lover, simply changing what kind of meat you eat can help you to eat more, for fewer calories. For example, a 6-ounce T-bone steak has over 200 calories more than either a sirloin or filet mignon of the same size, which means you could eat almost 9 ounces of the latter as opposed to the 6-ounce T-bone. (Although I wouldn't recommend eating all 9 ounces at once—that is a lot of meat!)

Sometimes it's the flavor you would like rather than a specific food. In the case of chocolate, for example, you could go for a handful of peanut M&M's (about ¼ cup) or eat almost a full cup of chocolate pudding. (That's almost four times more food!) You could also opt for some small Tootsie Rolls and eat ½ cup (double the amount).

You *could* eat...	OR Eat...
1 oz of chips (160 cal)	1.6 oz of pretzels (50% more!) or 2 1/2 cups of oil popped popcorn
3 cups of movie theatre popcorn (170 cal)	15 cups of air-popped popcorn
1/2 cup vanilla icecream (266 cal)	1 cup low fat icecream or 2 3/4 cups of non-fat icecream
1 croissant roll (270 cal)	3 1/2 dinner rolls
1 hamburger patty 75% lean (265 cal)	Almost 2 hamburger patties (95% lean)
1 cup whole milk (160 cal)	2 cups skim milk

Tool 4: Subtract by Addition

In seminars, I often ask people to tell me what comes to mind when they hear the word *diet*. Overwhelmingly, the responses include the following: hungry, eating rules, starving, carrots, brussels sprouts, not eating, and so on The emotions associated with this list usually include bitterness, resentment, hopelessness, and frustration.

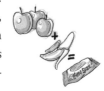

How would you like an eating plan that focuses on adding foods to your diet instead of subtracting foods?

Adding in certain foods, specifically fiber-rich foods, will help fill you up faster, feel full longer, and naturally combat overeating (not to mention the many other benefits that we receive by adding fiber into our diet, as discussed in Principle Two). The recommendations for fruits and vegetables (one of the best sources of fiber) used to be five servings a day of fruits and vegetables combined. The Dietary Guidelines for Americans has since increased the recommendations to 5 to 13 servings, combined, per day.[90]

Research supports this tool. Studies have shown that people who started meals at a restaurant with a low-calorie salad actually consumed up to 12 percent fewer calories during the course of the entire meal.[92–94]

When you feel the need to munch, go for vegetables or fruit, and you can't go wrong. You will actually end up consuming fewer calories when you eat more food.

A great dietitian and colleague of mine, Zonya Foco, gives great counsel on adding fruit to decrease your intake of sweets. She states that eating a piece of fruit and drinking a glass of water every four hours that you are awake will curb your sweet tooth and take away the gotta-have-sugar cravings. I've tried it. Many others have tried it. It works. Put it to the test. Try it today. Try it now. You will actually consume fewer calories by consuming more fruit.[95]

Three simple steps to increase fruits and vegetables in your diet

STEP 1 Buy fresh fruits and vegetables. (Buy in season for the best value. Try a local farmers' market, where you can often find lower prices and better flavor.)

STEP 2 When you get home, wash and cut the fruits and vegetables into portion sizes and put them in Ziploc bags (even sliced apples will stay good in Ziplocs for quite a while).

STEP 3 (the most important step): Put the baggies at eye level in the fridge. (In my perfect world, refrigerators would be built with the fruit and veggie bins right at eye level.)

How many times have you, with the best intentions, come home with a carload of fresh produce, dumped it in the fruit and veggie bins in the bottom of the fridge, closed the bins, and forgot about it until you opened the fridge a few weeks later to be smacked by some horrible smell? (Hey, I've done the same thing—don't be embarrassed.) Putting the produce at eye level, in ready-to-go baggies, makes it much more likely that you will grab it when you're wandering around the kitchen, aimlessly looking for something to munch.

If it helps, eat it with dip, have it with a little bit of peanut butter, sprinkle some cheese on it. Keep a big fruit bowl on the counter. Just eat it. Bulk up on fruits and vegetables.

Tool 5: Relax and Enjoy

It takes 20 minutes for the brain to interpret that the stomach is full. If you sit down to eat and start shoveling it in, you can inhale a lot of calories in those 20 minutes. The solution is simple. Stop. Relax. Enjoy the company.

One simple way to go about this is to physically force yourself to slow down. Set down the fork between every bite. Make yourself more aware of the act of eating. This seems almost too easy. Take it from someone who has tried it—it's not! It will drive you a little bit crazy at first to make yourself let go of the fork, set it down, and simply slow down. Try it. Try it today, at your next meal. It doesn't cost you a thing and can end up paying big dividends in weight loss. It also gives you the added benefit of really, truly savoring your food and enjoying the rich tastes and textures involved.

When you are eating with a group, take time to enjoy the atmosphere. Let yourself be there for the company, not the food. We are social animals, and a lot of our social engagements revolve around food. When you have eaten enough to feel satisfied, place a napkin over your plate as a signal to yourself that you are finished. This will help remind you when your fork mindlessly wanders to pick at your plate as the conversation flows. If you want to have some sort of hand-to-mouth contact, fill up on water instead.

Tool 6: Eat Offensively, Not Defensively

Do you eat to live or live to eat?

This question was posed by one of my professors and has stuck with me throughout the years as I reach for food throughout the day. The act of eating is, in fact, paramount to our survival. Eating is what fuels, energizes, and keeps our bodies alive. If we are not careful, however, eating can become much more than a means to survive—it can become all-consuming.

If you pause to think for even a few seconds when

you reach for that extra serving of chocolate cake or randomly wander into the pantry in the middle of the afternoon, you may discover that you are not there to relieve your hunger and to fuel your body.

This breakthrough of self-discovery can be the means to changing much about how you view your relationship to food and how much food you truly need for optimal health. It can help you shift your eating mentality from defense to offense.

You're an Offensive Eater If You:

- Often have plans for different meals.
- Strive each day to give your body the essential nutrients it needs for optimal health.
- Have a healthy relationship with food.
- View food as a friend to help you accomplish your life goals.
- Feel energized and renewed after meals and snacks.

You Might Be a Defensive Eater If You:

- Often have feelings of anger or regret after meals.

- Eat because of emotions rather than hunger.

- Seldom plan meals, resulting in quick, throw-together frozen or fast-food meals.

- View food as the "enemy," or categorize food as "good" and "bad."

- Have feelings of regret, leading to binging and the "I'll start tomorrow" mentality.

Tool 7: Eat Close to the Farm

No, you don't have to sell the house and head to the country. But that's where your food should come from.

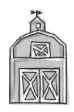 Do a quick test—run to your kitchen. Take a brief inventory. Do the bulk of the foods you eat come from a factory or a farm? For example: Does your orange supply come in the form of actual, off-the-tree oranges, orange juice, or orange soda? This should give you a quick check on where you stand right now.

The closer your food is to the farm, the healthier it will be. Always try to find fresh first. If not, move on frozen, then try canned (low salt), before heading to boxed.

Some experts simply recommend, "eat food." Yes,

this seems laughable and maybe a bit obvious, but try this: pick up a box of processed food in the store. Look at the ingredients. How many can you recognize?

No, you don't have to go through and throw out all of the processed food in your pantry, but do think about the ratio of processed foods that go into your body as compared to real food. If your ratio is extremely warped, simply take one step towards the farm. Offer your body one portion of real food at your next meal. Cut up an apple. Peel an orange. Snack on a banana. Chomp on some carrots. It doesn't matter what it is. Just one real food.

Once you have this in place, take one more step. Try, for just one meal during the week, to eat the entire meal based on real food. Think baby steps. You don't have to overhaul your pantry in one night, just start taking one step at a time towards the farm.

Tool 8: Use the Apple Test

" Life expectancy would grow by leaps and bounds if green vegetables smelled as good as bacon.**"**

—Doug Larson

When you find yourself standing in front of the fridge or the pantry, wondering what to eat, ask yourself this question: Would I eat an apple right now? (Or pick another fruit or vegetable that isn't quite what you would normally eat.) If you are truly hungry, then the answer will be yes, you would actually eat the apple. If not, the apple (or banana or carrot) won't sound good to you. You don't have to actually eat the apple, but this gives you a general sense of hunger versus appetite.

This also works for kids! When the kiddos are trying to stall bedtime, or trying to score some candy by claiming to be so hungry, simply ask them if they would like an apple, banana, and so on—again picking a food that they wouldn't normally crave or want. In my own house, this has worked like a charm. I simply offer my kids an orange. Sometimes they crinkle their nose and ask for some other treat-type food, but other times they will eat the orange or apple.

Tool 9: Drink Lots of Water

Yes, water works wonders in weight loss. Every function in your body requires water, including body-temperature regulation, digestion, metabolism, and nutrient transport.

Water also keeps your kidneys working well. This is important because without water, the kidneys start to shut down. Then the liver needs to overtake some of the kidney's duties and is no longer available for fat metabolism. This can lead to a decrease in fat breakdown and an increase in fat storage (not a good thing). Water also helps muscles to contract and release, especially during times of work or exercise, thus helping your body burn more calories.

Drinking water can actually help you get rid of extra water that your body may be holding on to. I know it seems counterintuitive when you are feeling bloated to drink even more water, but that is just what your body needs in order to let go of the excess water.

The majority of Americans walk around at any given time in varying states of dehydration. In fact, many times when you think you are hungry, your body actually just needs water. By the time you feel thirsty, your body is already dehydrated. Therefore thirst is not a good indicator of when you need water.

Dehydration can cause big problems with the body, such as dizziness, lack of concentration, headaches, slower metabolism, muscle weakness, and overheating, just to name a few.

The recommendations are to drink at least eight to ten cups of water a day. Sound like a lot to swallow? Well, it can be when you try to do it in big chunks.

The easiest way to increase your water intake is to invest in a water bottle and make it your best friend. Take it everywhere. Sip as often as you can. Make it a habit. Yes, you will need to take more potty breaks throughout the day, and yes, this is a good thing. It is a sign that your body is working. In fact, another good indicator of whether you are getting enough water is to look at the color of your urine. It should be a pale yellow.

Try this quick experiment: the next time you jump

in the car to run errands or to play car taxi, fill up a water bottle and then set it in your lap (or close to you in the car). Chances are, you will end up taking a bunch of little sips—while waiting at a light, waiting in a traffic jam, just to pass the time, and so on. Don't be surprised if you empty the entire water bottle in just one outing. That's water that you normally wouldn't have drunk had you not thought proactively and taken the water with you.

Tool 10: Keep a Food Journal

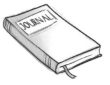

When I make the food journal assignment in my classes or with clients, I can usually see the participants visibly shudder. There is a reason for that. Deep down we all know that what we say we eat doesn't always match up with what actually goes into our mouths, and it's hard to be held accountable for our own actions, especially where food comes into play. We want the problem to be due to external circumstances and not our own hand-to-mouth issues.

In reality, food journaling has proven to be one of the most successful tools in weight loss and weight maintenance. Some studies even show that keeping a food journal can double the amount of weight loss.[96–100] Inconvenient? Yes. Frustrating? Yes. Will it help you reach your body goals? Absolutely. It does require you to be honest with yourself. If it goes in your mouth, it goes on the paper. It may even require a week of breaking out the measuring tools to make sure you are getting the portions correct.

Having to write everything down is one way to hold yourself accountable for and open your eyes to what you really put into your mouth. The first time I did this was for an assignment in college, and I was floored by what actually passed my lips during the course of a day. It was a pretty crazy, eye-opening experience!

There are many ways you can keep a journal: writing on a piece of paper, keeping a spreadsheet, or using a website or smartphone app. Find the one that works for you and start at your next meal. (See Appendix G for a food journal example.)

Tool 11: Use a Food-Group Checklist

If you know that writing down everything you eat won't work for you, here is another way to keep a running total of food by food group. Appendix H has a checklist for different levels of daily calories (1500, 1800, 2000). For example, a daily checklist for a 1500-calorie diet looks like this:

Carb (starch)						
Milk						
Fruit						
Meat						
Vegetable						
Fat						
Free						

Each box represents one serving of that food group. As you eat a food from the group, you simply check off the box. This way you can know at a glance what foods you have eaten during the day, and how much you can still eat.

Tool 12: Eat Mindfully

Much of our eating is done on autopilot. Especially when paired with other activities such as watching TV, reading, driving, and studying, the calories can pile up without our even noticing.

A whole book could be devoted to just this concept (and many are), but we will cover just the basics.

Give yourself permission to do nothing else but focus on the food in front of you.

Determine set times to eat and a set place where you will

eat, and let yourself simply enjoy the act of eating (instead of grabbing something on the way out the door or running through the drive-thru in between appointments). Let yourself truly delight in the taste, texture, aroma, and feel of the food. Allow yourself time to really enjoy eating as an activity in and of itself, not something to simply be choked down while on your way to another activity.

Eating is a pleasurable experience. Allow yourself to let go of the guilt and recapture the joy of eating.

If you want to take this tool one step further, try a little "mindful eating" experiment (I know, to many of you, this will not seem natural or even remotely what you are used to, but give it a try—you may surprise yourself.):

- Get one grape or raisin.
- Set it on a plate and study it.
- Think about where it came from, and all the steps that went into getting it from a seed in the ground to your plate.
- Put it in your hand and examine the color, shape, size, and aroma.
- Put it in your mouth (but don't bite yet!).
- Roll it around your mouth.
- Take note of how it feels in your mouth.
- Notice how your tongue explores the ridges of the raisin, or the smoothness of the grape.
- Fully feel all of the sides of the food as you move it around.
- Take just one bite.

- Let the taste wash over your whole mouth.
- Notice the aroma entering your nose to mix with the taste and intensify the sensation.
- Suck on it just a little to get more juice and taste out.
- Take your time to savor it completely before swallowing it. Linger as long as you can after each bite.
- Now, swallow and then simply remain still for a moment and notice the lingering sweetness in your mouth as you think about the contents that are now in your stomach, and what benefit the food will provide to your body.

Obviously, you don't have time to do this with every meal, but you'd be amazed just how much you can alter what you enjoy eating, simply by becoming more mindful of your mouthfuls.

Tool 13: Face Your Stuff, Don't Stuff Your Face

❝ If hunger is not the problem, then eating is not the solution.**❞**

—Author unknown

We eat for many reasons. Few of those actually have to do with hunger or health. For some reason, many of us have learned to hide our negative emotions or experiences. When those emotions come to the surface, we try to distract ourselves by reaching for some sort of comfort food.

One of my college professors outlined the cycle very well: you have a bad breakup with a significant other.

 You feel hurt, alone, or frustrated, but you don't quite know what to do about it. You see chips on the counter. You grab the bag and dig in, distracted by the act of eating. Before you know it, the whole bag is gone.

You are mad at yourself for eating the whole bag of chips, but at least it got your mind off the breakup for a while. The next time something frustrating happens, you look around to see what you can dig into to help keep you from having to face the emotions. And the cycle continues.

The solution to this is to allow yourself to feel emotions. There are no good or bad emotions. We all feel different emotions throughout the course of a day. It's okay to feel angry, or frustrated, or jealous. It's what we do in response to those emotions that can get us onto a slippery slope of emotional eating (or any other type of unhealthy behavior).

The key is to recognize the emotion before the food enters the mouth and then *stop*. Create a space for yourself to digest the emotion, instead of forcing yourself to digest the food. Think about it; feel it. Let yourself cry or scream or talk or walk or write. Whatever you need to do to let the emotion go. Let it in, let it out, let it go, and move on. Break the emotional tie to food.

If you are a visual person, cut out the stop sign in Appendix I (or download from all-diets-work.com) and hang it where you feel the most emotional triggers lead you to food, just to give you that added reminder to stop and feel the emotion before diving into the food.

Tool 14: Eat Breakfast

I know you've heard it before: breakfast is the most important meal of the day. This is true. Research has shown that right from the early stages of life, breakfast will help us perform better, think better, feel better, and look better.[23]

Eating breakfast will actually help you lose weight. Sounds crazy, right? But studies have proven this fact: eating breakfast is consistent with losing more weight, and with keeping weight off in the long run.[18, 101–8]

If you are not a breakfast eater, don't worry—it doesn't have to be the sit down country breakfast every morning. Anything in the morning helps.

QUICK BREAKFAST TIPS

Cold cereal—It's fast, it's cheap, and it's fortified with many vitamins and minerals to get you off to a great start.

Muffins—Bake ahead of time, freeze the batch, and then just pull out one or two the night before for a quick, on-the-go breakfast. (See Appendix J for some great, healthy, fill-you-up muffin recipes.)

Smoothies—A great way to start the day with a bunch of fruits (and vegetables). You can freeze the fruit for an even sweeter punch to the smoothie, and you won't have to add much ice. To save even more time, put enough fruit for one smoothie in a Ziploc in the freezer, then in the morning, just grab, blend, and go. (Smoothie recipes in Appendix J.)

Banana—Even grabbing a banana is better than nothing as you race through the kitchen on your way out the door.

Crockpot—Use a Crock-pot and put some oatmeal on to cook through the night. Come morning, it's ready for a quick and filling meal. Or try instant oatmeal, which is done in a matter of seconds, and then you can be on your way.

Tool 15: Take Control of the Restaurant Scene

Eating out is a fixture of modern life. Many of our cultural and social outings center around restaurants. Yet this is one of the biggest challenges for people who decide to change to a healthier way of eating.

If you do not eat out regularly and consider it a treat or special occasion, then allow yourself the freedom to order what you want, and enjoy it (making sure that you account for it and pay for it in calo- 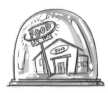 rie cash). One night, every once in a while, is not going to kill your overall nutrition plan.

On the other hand, if you are someone who eats out regularly, choose healthier options as often as you can. Here are some tips to help you manage both sit-down and fast-food restaurants:

WAYS TO NAVIGATE THE RESTAURANT

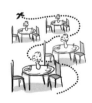

- Choose restaurants that have a variety of foods on the menu.

- If possible, go online before going out to find the nutritional analysis of your favorite menu choices. This will help you uncover the "hidden" calories and fat in some entrees. This will also help you to either make a healthier choice or to know how many calories are truly in the meal so that you can adjust the rest of the day accordingly.

- If going out with a friend, order one main dish and split it between the two of you.

- Right when the food comes, ask for a box. Divide it in half. Put half in the box, then enjoy the other half. Or better yet, ask the waiter to box half of it up when he plates it. Not only do you not have to worry about overeating at the restaurant, now you have lunch for tomorrow as well!

- Be bold (yet cordial) in asking for substitutions— have cream placed on the side, opt for the meat cooked in a different way, or substitute fresh fruit or vegetables for the side.

- Be careful in ordering dressing on the side: when dressing is brought this way, there is typically more dressing than is usually placed on the salad. If you dump it all on, you have defeated the purpose. Opt instead to dip the fork in the dressing before using it to pick up the salad. This gives you a taste of the dressing but doesn't overload you with fat or calories.

- When eating out with others, it doesn't count if you order the small salad, and then spend most of the meal "sampling" the plates of those around you. It may be hard to control the urge to grab some fries off of the kids' plates, but be honest with yourself.

Those calories do count, and they do add up.

- When eating in a group, speak up and be the first to order (one of the healthier options). You can set the stage and help other people also choose the healthier options when they see your example. (This way you will also eliminate the temptation to "snack" on potentially unhealthy options.)

- Don't be fooled by the "bottomless" drink. Not only are soda beverages extremely expensive, but studies have shown that when given a "bottomless" bowl (or cup), we lose our ability to determine how much we actually consume and end up drinking more than we think.[108]

WAYS TO NAVIGATE
THE FAST FOOD FURY

- Keep in mind that most fast-food places typically offer foods that are higher in fat, cholesterol, sodium, and calories and lower in vitamins, minerals, and fiber.

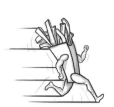

- Opt for baked, grilled or broiled when possible. At sandwich places, choose whole grain breads and make sure the high-calorie/fat sauces are used sparingly.

- When tempted to run through the drive-thru on the way home, ask yourself this simple question, "Is this truly faster than slapping together a sandwich at home?" Sometimes it is, but sometimes making something very simple at home is just as quick and much healthier (and cheaper too!).

- Avoid the urge to get soda pop. Ice water will help quench your thirst without loading you up with empty calories.

- The biggie sizes may seem like a great deal eco-nomically, but don't be fooled. More money will be saved in the long run by opting for the smaller size and preventing the many health problems that come with increased weight.

Tool 16: Shop Deliberately

How many times have you run into the grocery store for that one item and come out a hundred dollars later with a cart full of who-knows-what? Grocery stores offer a wide variety of items that can both help and hinder our health. Here are some general tips to help you navigate your way through the store:

1. Think perimeter.

The majority of healthy items are located around the perimeter of the store. Picture your favorite grocery store and think of where you would find fresh produce, fresh meat, dairy, and frozen foods. Chances are, you just mentally walked the perimeter of the building. When doing the shopping, try to stay on the perimeter as much as possible, only delving into the "catacombs" when you have to get something from your list. Even then, get in, get the item, and get out. Resist the urge to wander up and down the aisles. Not only will perimeter shopping create a healthier cart of items, but it will also save you money, by warding off impulse buying.

2. Make a list and stick to it.

This is especially helpful when paired with Tool 17: Plan Menus. Shopping from a list helps you save time and money.

3. Time it right.

Try to avoid shopping when tired, hungry, or in a hurry. Everything looks good when your stomach is growling, and you will almost certainly end up with more in the cart. Plus, you are much less likely to take the time to compare nutrition labels, check the ingredients list to make sure the "wheat bread" is really 100 percent whole wheat bread, and so on.

4. Leave the kids at home.

If you have children, I would also suggest that you go at a time when you can leave the kiddos with someone else so you don't have the constant temptation to give into the "Mommy, can I get . . . ?" requests.

Tool 17: Plan Menus

It's 5:00. Do you know what's for dinner? Gone are the days of spending all day in the kitchen simmering and cooking with whole foods. All too often, when the

time for eating draws near, we panic and reach for something quick and easy. Unfortunately, this also correlates with high calories, carbs, and fat. Taking a little bit of time weekly,

or even biweekly, to make a plan can reap huge long-term dividends in your goal of overall health.

Set a time frame (one week, two weeks, one month), and make a menu plan. (See Appendix K for a sample menu-planning sheet.) Your menu can be as simple as planning just main dishes for dinners, or as elaborate as planning out every part of every meal for each day in the plan. It's a good idea to jot down where the recipe can be found (if using a recipe) or even to attach the recipe to the menu sheet.

Once this is done, you can go through the list of ingredients, check the pantry, and, voila!, you suddenly have a complete grocery list.

The real beauty of planning ahead is this: you think with your head instead of with your stomach. Even jotting down an eating plan at night for the next day will help you focus more on what is healthy for your body instead of diving in to what is the easiest, most convenient thing to throw into your mouth throughout the day.

Tool 18: Eat to End Hunger, Not to Feel Full

" We never repent of having eaten too little.**"**

—Thomas Jefferson

Watch any baby, and you will see a natural mouth-to-stomach cue. Babies instinctively know when to turn away from food.

Somewhere between the "C'mon sweetie, just finish this last little bit of bottle" and the "You can't go play until you clean your plate" stages, kids learn to ignore their hunger cues and eat on a reward system instead. We have heard many versions of this. There's the guilt factor ("There are starving children in Africa—finish your plate!") and the bribe factor ("Nutritious before delicious—finish your vegetables if you want some chocolate cake."), which teaches us that healthy food is just something awful to be endured in order to get to the good stuff.

Give yourself permission to check out of the clean-plate club. Start by leaving just one spoonful on the plate. This little motion will allow you the chance to break from the have-to-finish mentality that has overridden the natural satiety centers in our brains.

This really takes being honest with yourself as you learn to listen to your body instead of your appetite (or your guilty inner voice about starving children). If it makes you feel better, box up the food and take it to the local food shelter—it will do much more good there than on your hips. If you absolutely cannot throw the unfinished portion away, simply put it in the fridge and use it at your next meal. You will actually be surprised at how much this can cut down on the food budget as you train yourself to eat just what feels good, instead of cleaning your plate.

Another great tactic is to eat small meals throughout the day instead of three big ones. The premise behind this is to eat smaller portions more frequently to stave off the grouchy/hungry phase, in which we often make poor food choices just to get something into our mouths.

Eating smaller meals to simply end the hunger will help you start to feel more energized and in tune with your body's natural hunger and need for nourishment, as opposed to what you want to taste on your tongue.

Tool 19: Stop the Stress

"*Stressed* spelled backward is desserts. Coincidence? I think not!**"**

—Author unknown

Give yourself a test: go through one day and count how many times you hear someone use the word *stress*. It's big and it affects all of us.

Any external or internal factor can be a stressor to someone. The body is hardwired to respond to stressful situations. In our ancestors' time, the stress response of the body literally saved lives. For example, when presented with a wild animal, the caveman had to respond by standing and fighting it off or running away quickly. This is where the stress response got the name "fight or flight."

The sympathetic nervous system triggers the release of two main hormones during this phase: adrenaline and cortisol. Adrenaline increases the heart rate and blood pressure, and helps to increase energy for activity. Cortisol works to increase glucose levels in the blood, and enhance the brain's intake of glucose, while decreasing bodily functions that are not essential during life-threatening situations, such as digestion, the immune system, the reproductive system, and the growth process.[110–11]

After the stress experience, the parasympathetic nervous system kicks in and helps bring the body functions back to normal.

Our modern-day stresses hardly entail meeting a wild animal face-to-face, or even events that require great physical work. Many times they happen while we are sitting at a desk, faced with a deadline, or sitting in a car in a traffic jam that is making us late for an important appointment.

Anything can cause stress, and different events cause different levels of stress for everyone: school, work, children, parents, traffic, wild animals charging at you, deadlines, and so on. Once you perceive a situation as stressful, however, the autonomic nervous system kicks in and releases the stress hormones. The sympathetic nervous system has the same response and releases extra glucose into the blood, which the body doesn't usually use up with either fighting or fleeing.

Over time, this can wreak havoc on the body.

EFFECTS OF LONG TERM STRESS[23, 110–11]

- Increased digestion problems
- Decreased immune system
- Decrease in restful sleep
- Increase in LDL
- Decrease in HDL
- Increase in blood glucose levels
- Increased risk for constipation
- Increased risk for heart problems
- Increase in blood pressure
- Increase in muscle tension
- Increase in weight
- Decrease in bone formation
- Increased hair loss
- Increase in jitters

Life will always be full of stressful events. That's the bad news. Here's the good news: you can change your response to stress. As Reverend Maureen Killoran says, "Stress is not what happens to us. It's our response to what happens. And response is something we can choose."

We have the ability to change how we view life events, and we can therefore increase our threshold to withstand stressful events. We can adapt the way we react to stress-triggering events in our lives. Stephen R. Covey in his book *The Seven Habits of Highly Effective People* explains a quote from Viktor Frankl (author of *Man's Search for Meaning*) as a stimulus-response cycle. Many times we feel we are locked into a certain behavior pattern in a given set of external stimuli:

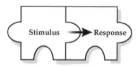

He explained, however, that in between the stimulus and response, there is a gap (however tiny it may seem) in which we have the power to choose how we will respond to the given stimuli. [112–13]

Really stop and think about this. There is great power and peace in that tiny gap. Regardless of what happens around you, you have the power to choose your own response. Think of how freeing this is! You are no longer dependent on the bar of chocolate to get you

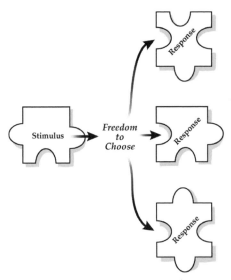

through the next staff meeting. You no longer have to reach for the donuts when the kids start acting up. You can choose. You can choose to react differently than you have in the past. You can choose to start acting differently today, right now. You have that power!

Another example is to picture a cup almost full of water. Think of that water as your wound-up insides. If you pour more water into the cup (a stressful event), it will overflow quickly (causing the fight-or-flight response). But if you can find ways to start with the cup almost empty, it would take many more stressful events before the cup overflows.

In this way, we can do things to help ourselves relax and lower the "water level" in our personal cup.

- Meditation
- Deep breathing
- Journal writing
- Exercise
- Performing acts of service
- Talking with a close friend
- Counseling
- Sleeping
- Listening to music
- Stretching
- Cleaning

Like the tools for weight loss in general, the tools for lowering stress are different for everyone. The key is to find what works for you and apply it whenever you feel the need to reach for food to de-stress.

Tool 20: Schedule Exercise

Exercise is not only one of the principles of weight loss, it is also a tool. In the Principles section, we discussed the whys of exercise. This section explains how to do it. Exercise is never something you will "have" time for. You must carve out time slots in your everyday life, and make exercise part of who you are.

When exercising, it is important to make sure that you are actually getting the benefits of exercise. That means that you want to make sure your body is working in the training zone. Use the following cues:

- **The talk test.** You should still be able to talk to your neighbor. If you can sing "The Star Spangled Banner," bump it up a notch. If you can't get in a "Hi, how are you?" bring it down a notch.

- **Sweat.** You should be working to the point that you are sweating. A Sunday stroll is nice, but it doesn't count toward the true exercise time.

- **Heart rate.** You should feel your heart beating pretty hard. If you are a numbers person, here is a quick guide to calculate your target heart rate, per minute: Subtract your age from 220, then multiply that number by 0.6 to find the low end and by 0.85 to find the high end. Your heart rate should be within this range for a one-minute pulse check. If you want to check your pulse for just 10 seconds during exercise, divide each of those numbers by 6, and that will give you the range you want to shoot for during the workout.

220 - Age = _____ x 0.6 = _____ /6 = _____
(low end of 10 second count)

220 - Age = _____ x 0.85= _____ /6 = _____
(high end of 10 second count)

Example

A 40-year-old's target heart rate would look like this:

220 - 40 = 180 (maximum heart rate)

180 x 0.6 = 108 beats (60-second count)
or 108/6 = 18 beats (10-second count)

180 x 0.85 = 153 beats (60-second count)
or 153/6 = 25 beats (10-second count)

This person's target zone in a 10-second count would be 18–25 beats.

Time for a Pop Quiz

Question 1: What is the best type of exercise you can do?

When I ask this in seminars, I get myriad answers. It's actually a trick question. The best type of exercise you can do is the type of exercise you enjoy doing (or at least something you will do on a regular basis). For example, I have taught aerobics for almost 20 years. Give me a little bench, a couple cubic feet, throw in some music, and I can happily exercise for a few hours. Tell me to get outside and run two miles, and I would much rather clean my toilets. True story. All of you runners out there, I admire you—I love that you have found what works for you. Running does not work for me, but I have found what does. Get rid of the guilt of not following the exercise routine that has helped your neighbor Nancy shed 35 pounds, and find what works for you.

Question 2: What is the best time for you to exercise?

Are you sensing a pattern? Again, the best time for you to exercise is the time that you can make it fit. Make an appointment with yourself, and write it in pen. Give yourself permission to tell people, "I'm sorry, I have an appointment at that time—I can't do x, y, or z for you." Yes, daily exercise is that important. Make that appointment whenever you can do it on a regular basis and stick to it. If you are not a morning person, don't set the goal to get up at 4:30 and run five miles. That will last as long as it takes to push "snooze" on your alarm. Carve out slots in the day in which you know you will be able to build a habit of exercise and let it become a part of who you are.

If you can't find a continuous 60 minutes, you can get smaller sessions throughout the day, provided they increase the heart rate enough to give the benefits of exercise. As stated in Principle 4, studies have shown that people who exercised for 10-minute mini-sessions throughout the day saw the same benefits as those who did the full amount of exercise in one setting.[45, 62]

MINI-SESSION IDEAS AT WORK

- Park farther away from the office and walk.

- Get off one bus stop early and walk.

- Walk or bike to work.

- Take the stairs.

- Have a meeting on a different floor? Opt for the stairs instead of the elevator.

- Deliver things personally instead of intra-office mail or email.

- Use the restroom on a different floor.

- Trade your coffee break for a fitness break and take a quick power walk.

- Start an office walking group—plan a time and get a group together: morning, lunch hour, or after work, whatever works for you.

MINI-SESSION IDEAS AT HOME

- Walk as much as possible (to neighbors, church, and so on).

- Use the bathroom on a different floor.

- Take several small piles of clothes to laundry room (instead of one large load).

- Vacuum often. (Try dancing to music as you vacuum!)

- Banish the couch potato—hide the remote, lift weights, do sit ups, bicycle while watching TV.

- Make a goal to be up and moving during every commercial break (somewhere other than to the fridge and back!).

- Walk in the mall in bad weather. (Leave the purse at home if it is too tempting to spend while you are there).

- Revisit activities of youth. (Try sledding or snow-man building in the winter; run through the sprin-kler or hop on the trampoline in the summer).

- Turn off the "automatic" drive on the lawn mower.

> • Have a few "snow blower" free days of shoveling the driveway in the winter.
>
> • Plant and tend a garden.

No, these are not new, earth-shattering secrets. These little tips have been around for years. So long, in fact, that at seminars, people can usually quote these to me. The medical show *The Doctors* decided to put them to the test in January 2011. They had a staff member put on a calorie counter. Day one, she lived life as normal and logged a baseline of calories burned. Day two, she implemented as many of these "little extras" as was possible during the course of her day. At the end of day two, she had burned more than 700 extra calories. Seven hundred! Just by adding in the little extras all throughout her day. They really do work.

Tool 21: Don't Be a Garbage Disposal

" Your stomach shouldn't be a waste basket.**"**

—Author unknown

My brothers were blessed with incredible metabolisms in their youth. When I was younger and we would go out to eat, anyone who couldn't finish his or her dinner simply sent the dinner remnants to one of the "human disposals" to finish it up. These brothers could finish everyone's meals and still have room for more (yet they never seemed to gain a pound).

Have you ever found yourself clearing the dinner table and "sampling" the little ones' leftovers? It's not quite enough to warrant breaking out a container to store it in—after all, it wouldn't even make a full serving—so instead of dumping it down the drain, you stick it in your mouth. Your thought process may even be well intended ("I can't let this food go to waste, it's like throwing away money!"), but do this enough, and you have just eaten another full dinner's worth of calories by the time the dishes are finished.

> When I buy cookies I eat just four and throw the rest away. But first I spray them with Raid so I won't dig them out of the garbage later. Be careful, though, because that Raid really doesn't taste that bad."
>
> —Janette Barber

Resist the urge to pop those small bites into your mouth.

If you feel guilty about wasting the money, think about this—you may pay a little now by throwing away the food, but you will pay a whole lot more later to get rid of the food once it overloads your body's calorie load.

If the temptation is too great, enlist the help of others to clear the table and do the dishes. (Your significant other will love me when you tell them where that thought came from. That's okay, throw me under the bus—I'll take the blame on this one.) Store the food, scrape the plate into the trash, back away, or leave the room—whatever you need to do to give yourself the signal that you are not the disposal. Set a goal that when you arise from the dinner table, your feeding time is officially over.

Tool 22: Look Long, Step Small

At one to two pounds of weight loss per week, progress on this road to wellness can seem like a snail's pace. The trick to help you see the big picture is long-term vision. For example, if it's summertime, make a goal for how you would like to look come Christmas. If it's Christmas, set a goal for how you want to look come July 4th. Or even picture yourself one year later.

The next step is to remember that goal every single day, and then every day ask yourself, "What am I doing today that will help me reach my next-year self?" The time will pass. Next year (or next season) will come. When it does, one of two things will happen. You will either (1) be excited and proud of yourself for making all of the tiny daily (and even hourly) choices to reshape your body, and enjoy reaping the benefits, or (2) be frustrated that you're stuck with the same habits and the same body, knowing that you are now on the other side of the time frame with nothing to show for it.

One tiny example of the power of small steps is in portion control. Tiny portion variations may seem inconsequential, but lets look at how small changes can compile over a year:

If you normally eat one cup of ice cream twice a week, cut the portion down to ½ cup. You will lose five pounds in a year—without doing anything else.
Here's the breakdown:

- 1 cup serving of rich ice cream = 350 calories x 104 (twice a week for 52 weeks) = 36,400 calories/year
- ½ cup of ice cream = 175 calories x 104 = 18,200/year (5 pounds less!)

If you go more extreme and opt for low-fat or fat-free ice cream you can save even more:

- ½ cup low-fat ice cream = 115 calories x 104 = 11,960/year (7 pounds less)
- ½ cup fat-free ice cream = 95 calories x 104 = 9,880/year (8 pounds less)

Other small steps you can take:

- If you trade one 12-ounce can of soda pop a day for water, you will drop 15½ pounds in just one year without doing anything else. If you drink 20 ounces a day and change that size for water, you will drop a whopping 26 pounds. Again, that is without doing anything else.
- If you are a donut-a-day person, the simple act of changing the donut to a granola bar will help you drop 20 pounds in one year.
- If you eat chips (3 ounces) every night while

watching TV, and simply change it for popcorn (5 cups light microwave popped), you could drop a whopping 28 pounds in one year (while eating more food!).

Small changes really do add up to big dividends in the weight-loss journey!

Tool 23: Use the Buddy System

Studies support the need for buddies, especially in the war on weight. In one study comparing two different types of diets, both were effective in producing weight loss—with a support system in place. Without a support system, the weight loss in both was very minimal (a few pounds after two years).[114] Again, it's not the specific diet that is the reason for the loss (although in this study, the people who followed the vegan diet with support did lose more than those on the standard diet with support), the biggest difference is going at the diet alone versus having a buddy.

There is something about having to be accountable to someone that can kick you into gear. It can be as formal as meeting with a registered dietitian weekly, biweekly, or monthly, joining a weight-loss support group, or simply partnering up with a friend or relative to help keep you accountable.

Tool 24: Weigh In Weekly

❝In the Middle Ages, they had guillotines, stretch racks, whips and chains. Nowadays, we have a much more effective torture device called the bathroom scale.❞

—Stephen Phillips

This one is a touchy subject with many people. For a while I advised all of my clients to throw away their scales and just monitor their changing body shape. I saw so many people live and die by that number on the scale, and it sent them to a bad place emotionally every time they stepped on the scale.

For many people, it is extremely frustrating to work so hard all week and then only have a few ounces of difference to show for it (or worse, to see an increase of a pound). In fact, the same body can differ in weight by as much as five  pounds in any given day, due to a variety of factors (hydration status, sweating from exercise, meals, or even nursing or menstruation for women).

Now, however, I guardedly advise people to weigh in weekly. The scale can be a powerful tool to help with weight loss and weight maintenance.[115–16] It can help you catch little moments of regain before they turn into a new pattern of upward (and consequently outward) momentum (which in the world of weight control is not a good thing).

This tool requires you to really know yourself emotionally. If you know this would help motivate you and keep you on schedule, then great, break out that scale. If you know that your day/week/month would be ruined by the numbers you see, and if instead of motivating you, it sends you into the mindset of "why even try?" as you dive into the closest bag of Oreos, then this is not the tool for you.

If you decide to use a scale, the most effective way to do so is to weigh yourself at the same time each week, with the same clothes on (or none at all).

Tool 25: Use Meal Replacements

Like weighing in, this tool won't work for everyone, but it does have its place. Meal replacements can be anything from shakes, to frozen meals, to meals delivered to your house. Although more expensive than other alternatives, if you don't have the time to prepare healthy meals, this may be a viable option for you. The beauty of these meals is that they are portioned for you, so then take the guesswork out of deciding how much is a serving. It also saves time in planning and cooking your own meals. If you opt for the shake replacement, you must remember that the drink is the meal, not just the drink.

WHAT'S IN YOUR TOOLBOX

The best weight-loss solution for you is the one you build yourself. Here are stories of real people and the tools they have used to change their lifestyles, lose weight, and build healthy bodies. For more success stories (and to add your own) go to all-diets-work.com.

Saved by the Beach

Kevin Buman, 35

As long as I can remember, I always considered myself overweight. As a boy I was often referred to as "husky." This term was somehow more socially acceptable when talking about a child. But I knew when someone was trying to be protective of my feelings.

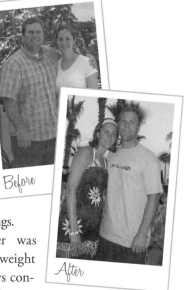

Before

After

Because my mother was constantly fighting a weight battle herself, I was always conscious about food. In our house, we never had sugary cereals or full-fat anything. Bread was always whole grain, meat was always lean, and there was never any candy. The thought was that if we didn't have "unhealthy" choices in the house, we would never eat them. However, when confronted with different (and, frankly, more appealing) choices while outside the home, I ate them—and a lot of them.

In the fall of 2006, I moved to a new state with my young family. My son was five years old, and my daughter was just about to turn two. I weighed about 70 pounds above my normal BMI range. With long hours of work and the stress of the move, I gained another 15 pounds in four months.

My turning point came in 2007, while looking at photos of my brother's recent beach wedding in Cancún. I was shocked at the way I looked. I was very sad. I finally realized that I needed to do something about my weight, but I had tried so many times before and nothing worked. I was uncomfortable in my own skin and didn't know what to do to fix it.

My mother, understanding my frustration, offered to pay to get me started in the Weight Watchers program. I decided to take her up on it and joined Weight Watchers in March of 2007, weighing 269 pounds.

My Toolbox

Tool 10: Keep a Food Journal

The Weight Watchers program gave me a new perspective on food. I learned that I must take responsibility for what I eat and be accountable. It wasn't about starving myself and always feeling hungry but more about keeping track of what I do eat and eating the right foods. In the past, I would eat anything, regardless of calories, fat, or any other nutritional indicator.

Tool 3: Eat by Volume

My perception of weight loss wasn't about eating different food but rather about eating less food. I thought losing weight and eating healthily meant only one cheeseburger at McDonald's instead of two or three and ordering the medium fries instead of the large. I have since come to understand that although portion control is certainly important, the type of food you eat is more important.

Tool 22: Schedule Exercise and Tool 23: Use the Buddy System

After I lost about 40 pounds, I thought I would start to include an exercise routine to see if I could increase my weight-loss results. I found a friend who liked to run and was willing to slow down his pace while I got started. I quickly realized that I enjoyed running. What I loved most was the social aspect of running and the feeling that I got when I was done. I would run early in the morning before work, and that seemed to make me feel better about myself for the rest of the day.

Between March 2007 and June 2008, I lost 82 pounds. Since that time, I have maintained my weight (within seven pounds). By finally changing my attitude toward food, I hope I am now setting an example for my children that will positively effect their own eating habits and consequently their own body images.

Treats, Tennis, and Teenagers

Ann Eberhard, 42

Five years ago, I was diagnosed with a medical condition that required surgery. To be eligible for the surgery, I had to lose at least 30 pounds in less than three months. With the help of a dietitian, I lost 37 pounds before the surgery.

Before

It was a miserable experience, which I don't recommend to anyone. I felt like I was always hungry and always exercising.

After the surgery was over and I was able to eat normally again, I decided I did not want to gain the weight back. Now I had to figure out how I was going to keep the weight off. I knew I did not want to always be hungry. And I didn't want to spend my life denying myself the things that I loved. Remembering what the dietitian taught me about burning more calories than I ate, I decided to eat healthy and exercise but allow myself some treats.

My Toolbox

Tool 20: Schedule Exercise

If I split my hour of exercise into two sessions—morning and evening—I seem to be able to more easily keep the weight off. I also decided to find an exercise that I love to do, so it would be fun. Tennis was one of my answers. I love it! Another answer was to do activities with my children. They have to go on their paper routes; I walk with them. They go sledding, so do I. My children make me laugh and keep me focused on fun, not exercise.

Tool 2: Slendersize

I learned that it is okay to have chocolate—I just cut my portions way down. When I did this, I realized that a small portion of dessert still satisfies me, especially if I eat it slowly so I finish with everyone else. I also learned that portion size is everything. I like having seconds if everyone else is, so I start with small firsts and have small seconds. I find I am satisfied and happy.

Tool 9: Drink Lots of Water

If I remember to drink water first, I eat less.

Tool 22: Look Long, Step Small

I can't do dramatic things, but I can do small things. And small things have made the difference for me.

Muscle Woman

Dawn Caccavale, 38

All my life I had been athletic and skinny; I could eat whatever I wanted and my weight pretty much stayed the same. (Yes, I know, annoying.)

Then everything changed. I had my first child at 35 and my second at 37 and ballooned from 130 pounds to 210 pounds, on a five-foot-four frame. I was so big that I didn't even know what size I was—I just wore elastic-waist pants and large maternity T-shirts for a year.

Before

After

I decided I was far too vain to be that huge and joined a gym. I had no idea where to start, so I did what most people do and I got on the treadmill and stopped eating. It worked a little, but I was super annoyed all the time because I was so hungry, plus I was still flabby. It was time for some research.

My Toolbox

Tool 5: Addition by Subtraction

I called an ex-body builder I knew and picked his brain. Then I got started. I did eat less—less junk food. But I bumped my veggies, protein, and water way up.

Tool 20: Schedule Exercise

My biggest change was with my cardio regimen. I went from 160 minutes a week to none. Yup. The only cardiovascular workout I got was what I experienced in class—weight lifting class.

My friend told me I should lift weights at least four times a week, preferably six. He also said I needed to lift as heavy as I could. Since I'm one of those people that needs to be stuck in a class for an hour to really get a workout, I took power cut, kettle bells, pilates, and yoga classes. After six months, here I am, 130 pounds, eating whatever I want again (within reason).

I learned that gaining muscle mass helps burn calories and makes you look hot in your pants again. Your non-elastic pants. Oh, and I don't look like Burt the ex-body builder, I look like Tara Stiles the yoga instructor. So don't worry ladies! Pick up the (heavy) weights and lose the flab—your skinny jeans miss you.

Big Winner

Heather Lee, 40

It had been a very long time since I was thin, or even an average weight for my height. However, when my fourth child was born, complications with the C-section left me with chronic pain. I dealt with the pain by eating comfort food—and lots of it.

After about a year, I had gained 25 pounds, in

addition to the pregnancy weight I hadn't lost. I decided to put some effort into losing weight, and with a little exercise, I lost 10 pounds over the next six months. Then winter set in, and exercise ceased.

My Toolbox

Tool 23: Use the Buddy System

When spring came, my family decided to have a Biggest Loser contest. Each person contributed 50 dollars in at the beginning and then 5 dollars each month. The overall winner would take the big pot, and each month the biggest loser took home the monthly pot.

After

Our first weigh-in was that night after a huge meal (including two desserts). Getting on that scale in front of my entire family was probably one of the most embarrassing experiences of my entire life. I was far from being the heaviest, but it was still so humiliating for my family to know how heavy I'd become. That started my true weight-loss journey.

The next six months had some ups and downs, but

overall I lost 35 pounds and won the whole competition. It was an amazing experience for me.

Tool 4: Subtract by Addition

One of the most effective things I did was to drink a glass of water and eat a piece of fruit every four hours while I was awake to cut down on my sugar cravings. I was amazed how well this worked. If I waited until I was dying for a candy bar, a banana didn't cut it. But if I kept to the routine, it worked really well.

Tool 2: Slendersize

Another big change was my portion sizes. I started paying attention to how much food I was putting on my plate. When I slowed down and paid attention, I found I could eat much less and still feel satisfied. This worked great when eating out as well. I could still have the hamburger that I love, but an 89-cent burger filled me up just fine; I didn't need the six-dollar burger. I shared my fries with my girls instead of eating them all myself. I didn't cut out dessert all the time. If I didn't treat myself sometimes, I knew I'd never succeed.

Tool 3: Eat By Volume

Snacking is huge in my world, and I'm amazed how filling a handful of almonds in the afternoon can be. If I really crave chips, I can trick myself by eating a few chips then a handful of nuts, which fills me up and make me feel satisfied.

Tool 20: Schedule Exercise

Probably the biggest secret to my weight loss was exercise. I'd been running/walking around 20 to 30 minutes a day. When I upped that amount to 45 to 60 minutes a day it made a huge difference. How did I make this happen? I watched the entire series of *Lost* on the treadmill. It's amazing how much more motivating it is to exercise when you are dying to find out what is going to happen next on that mysterious island in the middle of nowhere.

I'm now watching *24* and it does the same thing. You can't imagine the adrenaline rush Jack Bauer in a crisis can bring to the treadmill. Several times, I have walked at least a quarter of a mile more than I planned because I was caught up in the story.

More than a year after earning my new status as the biggest loser, I'm still wearing sizes 6 and 8. I'm wearing medium-size shirts. I have great muscle definition, and I feel better than I have in a long time. That is a big win.

Facing My Stuff

Robin Conner, 31

I started seeing food as something bad when I was around seven or eight. My health-conscious mother forbade sugar in the house. Eating out was almost unheard of.

When sugar or not-so-healthy food was around, (special occasions, birthdays and holidays) I lusted after

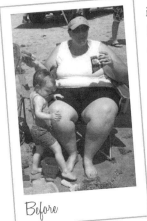

Before

it, craved it, thought about it, and thought about how to obtain more until it was gone. I would sneak and hide food, and then when I thought I was alone, I'd go eat it. When friends asked me to stay for dinner, I would in a heartbeat. Then I'd go home and eat dinner there as well.

Food was starting to fill a hole inside me. It made me feel full inside. It kept me company. It was always there and never left me.

I stayed pretty average in size during my teenage years. I was bigger than my friends, but I was by no means obese.

Then came the magical day when I moved out on my own and made my own money. I bought and hoarded anything fried, filled with sugar, and bad for me. I ate and ate and ate until I was literally sick. Then I'd go to bed, wake up, and do it all over again. I was eating at fast-food joints multiple times a week and sometimes several times

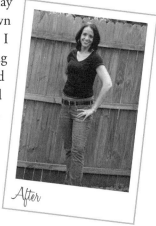

After

a day. Sugar was everywhere in my house, and I ate it constantly—especially chocolate. I could down a dozen glazed Krispy Kreme donuts in less than 20 minutes flat. It felt awesome.

At age 18, I weighed 170 pounds. By 20, I was already 250 pounds. I started having children. After our fourth child was born, I was 29 years old and a whopping 323 pounds.

At night, when the kids were in bed, it was my time. I would load up my arms with chips, cookies, and ice cream, and head to the couch for emotional eating nirvana. This was my routine for ten years. I looked forward to it, daydreaming about what I would binge on that night.

In February 2010, the year I would turn 30, something snapped in my brain. I realized, "This is my life. The only person I'm rebelling against is myself. The only person I'm hurting is myself. I am in control of my life. Now, what am I going to do about it?"

My Toolbox

Tool 20: Schedule Exercise

I got a gym membership. Now, after the kids went to bed, I started going to the gym instead of sitting on the couch. The gym hurt. After three minutes on the elliptical machine, I was dying to get off. I hated it. I hated seeing all the skinny girls and muscular men strut around. I hated seeing myself in the mirror at the gym. I was huge.

But I kept going. Soon my cardio went from 20 minutes to an hour. And it actually felt good. I added weight lifting. Soon, my energy was through the roof, and I was losing weight.

Tool 13: Face Your Stuff, Don't Stuff Your Face

After the two-week mark, where I had always quit before, I found myself binging on potato chips in one hand and Oreos with peanut butter spread on them. What was I doing? Why was I doing this? What need is this filling?

I started to pay close attention to when I went out of control and what was happening at that exact moment.

I identified my triggers: disobedient children, schedule fluctuations, a busy workload, and other stressful moments. Instead of facing the moment head-on and dealing with the accompanying feelings and emotions, I would stuff my face.

I decided to get comfortable with being uncomfortable—staying in the moment and letting myself feel everything, as unbearable as it was. I stopped running away from life. Like a bad boyfriend, I had to literally break up with food.

What was the side effect to my new choices? Weight loss. This was not a diet. This was not a special exercise regimen. This was me gaining control of my life and my emotions, and the end result was weight loss.

Do I ever eat ice cream, cake, brownies, french fries, or hamburgers? Heck yes, I do. Do I binge on them till

I'm in a food-induced coma? No. Do I still mess up? All the time. But the key to my success is to always move forward. I will never let emotional eating conquer my life again.

Back to Softball

Chad Bickel, 48

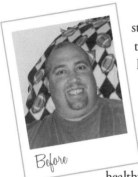

Before

My journey to a healthy lifestyle started in 2006, when my doctor told me that my blood pressure was high and I needed medication. She also said that my blood sugar and cholesterol were high and I could become diabetic if I did not lose weight. The numbers confirmed what I already knew: I wasn't healthy, and I didn't feel good. I had such a low energy level and chest pain when walking up a flight of stairs. I even had to stop playing softball.

In January of 2007, I joined a gym. I was determined to lose the weight and stick to it no matter what. My inspiration came from the show *The Biggest Loser*. I thought if they could do it, so could I.

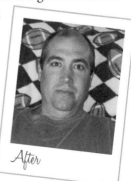

After

My Toolbox

Tool 2: Slendersize

I bought a food scale and weighed out the portions, so I knew exactly how many calories were going in my mouth.

Tool 10: Keep a Food Journal

I started using the Jillian Michaels weight-loss program online to keep a food diary and track my calories.

Tool 20: Schedule Exercise

My workout routine consisted of 20 minutes of cardio and 30 minutes of lifting weights. I did that six days a week and sometimes twice a day.

By February of 2007, I had already lost 30 pounds I decided to hire a personal trainer to help me maximize my workout. I was determined not to fail. My routine changed to forty-five minutes of cardio and 60 minutes of weights. By the summer of 2007, I had lost 100 pounds.

Four and a half years later, I am now maintaining a healthy weight, off my blood pressure pills. I am back to playing softball. Determination was the key to my success.

Breakfast Shmeakfast

Dolores Causler, 66

I was 28 years old and knee-deep in toddlers. At 200 pounds, I wasn't keeping up with them, and I wasn't keeping up with my husband, who was very fit.

After several half-hearted attempts to reform, I decided I needed to make a commitment and get in shape.

My Toolbox

Tool 20: Schedule Exercise

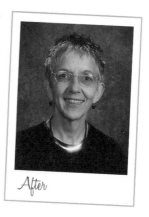

After

I had accompanied a friend to the gym a few times, but I didn't like to work out, and quickly fizzled. However, I finally decided to make a commitment and join a gym. I still didn't like going, but I went. And I kept going. I continued to dread going to the gym until I brainwashed myself into actually enjoying the classes. I was so successful at tricking myself into it that I now actually teach senior fitness classes at the gym—and I love it!

Not Tool 14: Eat Breakfast

For years, I ate breakfast because I was supposed to—it's the "most important meal of the day." But I never really feel hungry in the morning. So I decided to skip it. I would go to school and teach a full load of classes and then eat lunch, my first meal of the day, at the same time as my students. Sometimes I'd have some fruit between classes. I've just found that for me, this is the best way to keep my daily calorie intake at the right level.

Tool 22: Look Long, Think Small

When I first started trying to lose weight, I tried all sorts of diets: the cabbage soup diet, the Mayo Clinic diet, etc. At the school where I teach, we had several weight-loss contests, where we'd pool our money and reward the people who lost the most weight. I always won part of the pot because I was disciplined enough. But then I'd gain it right back. It wasn't until I changed my daily habits in small ways that I was able to maintain the weight loss.

Tool 4: Subtract by Addition

I love fruit. My mother always had fruit in the house, and it was always available. So one thing that worked to control my eating habits was to always make sure I had fruit and a bag of carrots at my desk at school. Sometimes that meant stopping at the store on the way to work. Fruit and vegetables became my trademark at school. Kids would tease me about it, and I'd share with them when they came to talk to me after school. For me, part of the appeal of fruit is the chewing factor—carrots really do it for me.

Tool 1: Pay Cash for Your Calories

When I know I'm going to want a treat, I don't deprive myself of the treat—I just plan ahead. If I'm planning to eat popcorn at the movies, I'll limit my calories at dinner. If I'm going to get pie with friends, I order just pie, not dinner. If I have a big meal coming up, like Thanksgiving, I plan ahead and consume fewer calories a few days before, eating lots of fruit and drinking plenty of water.

I love desserts and sweets and don't want to give them up. I don't eat them daily. I'm in control.

For the last 15 to 20 years, I have weighed under 140 pounds. I used to be motivated by wanting to look better. Now I don't care what I look like—when you get to be my age, droopiness is inevitable. What motivates me is waking up and feeling good, walking fast, and keeping up with my husband. Some women and men in my age group can barely bend over. They can't think about going for a mile hike along the river. I'm grateful for my good health every day.

APPENDIX

Appendix A: Carbohydrates

Appendix B: Protein

Appendix C: Fats

Appendix D: Vitamins and Minerals

Appendix E: Basal Metabolic Rate

Appendix F: Calorie Dollars

Appendix G: Food Diary Example

Appendix H: Food Group Checklist

Appendix I: Stop Sign

Appendix J: Recipes

Appendix K: Meal-Planning Worksheet

Appendix A: Carbohydrates

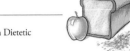

(Adapted from references 21-23 and the American Dietetic
Association www.eatright.org)

FUNCTIONS:
➡ Provides energy for the body. Each gram of carbohydrate supplies
   4 calories.
➡ The only source of energy for the brain.
➡ In fiber form, carbohydrates can decrease risk for cancer and can
   decrease cholesterol (See see following page for food sources of fiber.).

RECOMMENDATIONS:
About 45-65% of total calories should come from carbohydrates.
Example: A 2,000-calorie diet should include 248-358 g of carbohydrates.

FOOD SOURCES:
Bread, grain, pasta, popcorn, rice, cereal, milk, fruits, vegetables.
Always try to choose whole grains (think brown), which provide complex
carbohydrates — the best form of carbohydrates.

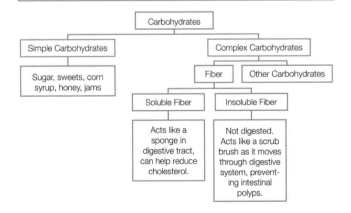

ESTIMATED FIBER CONTENT OF FOODS*

(Compiled from sources 22-25, 117):

Great Source (7-18+gm):
→ All Bran Cereal
→ Baked Beans
→ Bran Buds
→ Broccoli (cooked, ¾ cup)
→ Butter Beans
→ Dried Figs
→ Fiber One Cereal
→ Great Northern Beans
→ High-Bran Bread
→ Kidney Beans
→ Navy Beans
→ Okra
→ Peas (green, fresh with pods)
→ Spinach (1/2 cup cooked)

Very Good Source (5-6 gm):
→ Benefit Cereal
→ Black Beans
→ Black-Eyed Peas
→ Bran Meal
→ Brown Rice
→ Brussel Sprouts
→ Guava
→ Lentils
→ Pinto Beans
→ Pumpernickle Bread
→ Raisin Bran Cereal
→ Turnips
→ White Potato
→ Whole Wheat Bread
→ Whole Wheat Spinach Noodles
→ Yams

ESTIMATED FIBER CONTENT OF FOODS (CONT.)

Good Source (2-4 gm):

- Apples
- Apricots
- Artichokes
- Beets
- Blackberries
- Bran Muffins
- Broccoli (raw)
- Carrots
- Chick Peas
- Cranberries
- Egg Plant
- Fresh Figs
- Grits
- Lima Beans
- Oatmeal
- Parsnips
- Peach
- Pears
- Plums
- Popcorn
- Prunes
- Rye Bread
- Sliced Almonds
- Strawberries
- Sweet Potato
- Whole Wheat Bread Crumbs
- Whole Wheat Egg Noodles

*Important note: It is difficult to find the exact fiber content in many foods (including fruits and vegetables) due to the complexity of the food. Because of this, the estimated amount of fiber per serving may vary between different sources. The author has used the most commonly quoted values for these charts.

**psst: did you notice that most beans are really high in fiber? Want a sneaky way to add fiber in a way that everyone loves? Simply substitute pureed beans for oil in cake and muffin recipes (light beans in light colored cakes, dark or light beans in chocolate cakes, cup for cup in place of oil). It works, I promise! This was a trick I learned from the blog www.Everydayfoodstorage.net a while ago and I have been using it ever since. Shh, don't tell my husband or kids — they still have no idea…

Appendix B: Protein

(Adapted from references 21-23 and the American Dietetic Association www.eatright.org)

FUNCTIONS:

- ➡ Provides energy for the body. Each gram of protein provides 4 calories.
- ➡ Builds muscles, organs, tissues, and cells.
- ➡ Helps body heal wounds.
- ➡ Aids in immune system function.

RECOMMENDATIONS:
Consume .8 g of protein each day for each kilogram of body weight.
You should get about 10-15% of your calories from protein.
Example: A 160 lb woman weighs 72.5 kg. 72.5 kg x .8 =
58 g protein per day

FOOD SOURCES:

Meat, dairy, eggs, nuts, peanut butter,
some cereals, some vegetables (beans).

Appendix C: Fats

Types of Fat:

Trans Fatty Acid

Saturated Fatty Acid

Monounsaturated Fatty Acid

Polyunsaturated Fatty Acid

Appendix D: Vitamins and Minerals

(Adapted from references 21-23 and the American Dietetic Association www.eatright.org)

Fat Soluble Vitamins (A, D, E, K):

Vitamin A

FUNCTIONS:
→ Cell function
→ Growth and development
→ Immune functions
→ Reproduction health
→ Vision

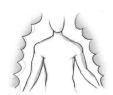

DAILY RECOMMENDATIONS

(measured in retinol activity equivalents, RAEs):
Infants and young children: 400-500 RAE
Children and teens: 600-900 RAE
Adults: 700-900 RAE
Pregnant: 750-770 RAE
Lactating: 1200-1300 RAE

FOOD SOURCES:
Turkey, 1 cup: 15,534 RAE
Sweet potato, 1 small: 7,374 RAE
Carrots, raw, 1 cup: 5,553 RAE
Spinach, cooked, 1 cup: 6,882 RAE
Butternut squash, 1 cup: 2,406 RAE
Mixed veggies, 1 cup: 2,337 RAE
Apricots, canned, 1 cup: 1,329 RAE
Cantaloupe, 1 cup: 1,625 RAE
Broccoli, cooked, 1 cup: 1,625 RAE
Brussel sprouts, 1 cup: 430 RAE
Tomatoes, 1 cup: 450 RAE
Peaches, canned, 1 cup: 283 RAE

Vitamin D

The body can build Vitamin D through exposure to the sun, although sunscreen prevents absorption. When you're not routinely exposed to the sun without sunscreen, be sure to consume adequate amounts of Vitamin D in your diet.

FUNCTIONS:
➡ Helps maintain calcium levels
➡ Increases calcium and phosphorus absorption in intestine
➡ Helps bones re-absorb calcium
➡ Works in kidneys to decrease calcium loss in the urine

DAILY RECOMMENDATIONS:
Infants to young adults: 5mcg (200 international units (IU))
Adults: 5-15mcg (200-600 IU)
Adults 51-70 years: 10mcg (400 IU)
Adults 70+: 15mcg (600 IU)

FOOD SOURCES:
Herring, 1 ounce: 6.6mcg (461 IU)
Salmon, 1 ounce: 2.1mcg (130 IU)
Cod liver oil, 1 tablespoon: 33mcg (1350 IU)
Fortified Milk, 1 cup: 2.5mcg (100 IU)
Sardines, canned, 1 ounce: .7mcg (187 IU)
Egg yolk: .6mcg (20 IU)
Fortified breakfast cereal, 1 cup: .5-2.5mcg (20-100 IU)

Vitamin E

FUNCTIONS:
→ antioxidant
→ cell membrane structure

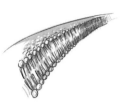

DAILY RECOMMENDATIONS:
Infants: 4-5mg
Young children: 6-7mg
Older children and teens: 11-15mg
Adults: 15mg
Pregnant: 15mg
Breastfeeding: 19mg

SOURCES (mostly fortified cereals and plant oils,

such as salad oil, margarine, and shortening):
Raisin bran, 1 cup: 13.50mg
Almonds, ¼ cup: 9.4mg

Sunflower oil, 1 tablespoon: 5.59mg
Mixed nuts, 1 ounce: 3.10mg
Canola oil, 1 tablespoon: 2.39mg
Asparagus, 1 cup: 2.16mg
Apricots, canned, ½ cup: 1.55mg
Margarine, 1 tablespoon: 1.27mg
Baked beans, 1 cup: .25mg

Vitamin K

FUNCTIONS:
➡ blood clotting
➡ bone formation and health
➡ regulation of some enzymes

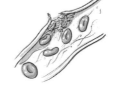

DAILY RECOMMENDATIONS:
Infants: 2.0-2.5mcg
Children to teens: 30-75mcg
Adults: 90-120mcg

FOOD SOURCES:
Spinach, cooked, 1 cup: 1027mcg
Broccoli, cooked, 1 cup: 220mcg
Asparagus, cooked, 1 cup: 144mcg
Cabbage, cooked, 1 cup: 75mcg
Beet greens, cooked, ½ cup: 348mcg
Collard greens, cooked, ½ cup: 418mcg
Grapes, 1 cup: 23mcg
Cucumber, raw: 49mcg
Kale, cooked ½ cup: 531mcg
Kiwi, medium: 30mcg
Prunes, stewed, 1 cup: 65mcg
Strawberries, sliced, 1 cup: 23mcg
Swiss chard, cooked, ½ cup: 286mcg
Tuna canned, 3 ounces: 37mcg

Common Water Soluble Vitamins (B2, B12, Folate, C)

Vitamin B2 (riboflavin)

FUNCTIONS:
➙ Helps metabolize carbohydrates, fats, and protein
➙ Helps protect the cells by supporting antioxidants

DAILY RECOMMENDATIONS:
All ages: between .3 and 1.6 mg

FOOD SOURCES:
Beef liver, 3 ounces: 2.91mg
Fortified cereal, 1 serving: up to 1.7mg
Milk, 1 cup: .45mg
Cottage cheese, 1 cup: .37mg
Hamburger, lean, 3.5 ounces: .21mg
Cheese, 1 ounce: .1 mg
Banana: .09 mg

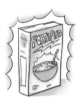

Vitamin B12

FUNCTIONS:
➡ Aids in amino acid metabolism
➡ Aids normal functioning of all cells,
   but especially GI tract, bone marrow,
   and nervous tissue

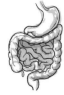

DAILY RECOMMENDATIONS:
All Ages: .4-2.8mcg
Teens: 2.4mcg
Pregnant: 2.6mcg
Breastfeeding: 2.8mcg

FOOD SOURCES:
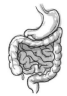
Liver, 3.5 ounces: 70.7mcg
Oysters, 6 medium: 16mcg
Crab, 3 ounces: 9.8mcg
Lamb chop, boneless, 3 ounces: 2.7mcg
Tuna, 3 ounces: 2.5mcg
Hamburger, lean, 3 ounces: 2.4mcg
Cottage cheese, 3 ounces: 1.6mcg
Turkey, 3 ounces: 1.3mcg
Yogurt, with fruit, 8 ounces: 1.1mcg
Skim milk, 1 cup: 1.3mcg
Cereals, 1 serving: .5-6.0mcg

Folate (Folic Acid)

FUNCTIONS:
- ➡ Essential for new cell formations, especially in pregnancy
- ➡ Nervous system
- ➡ May protect against heart disease
- ➡ Synthesis and repair of DNA
- ➡ Helps in formation of red and white blood cells in bone marrow

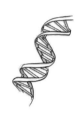

DAILY RECOMMENDATIONS:
Teens and adults: 400mcg
Pregnant: 600mcg
Breastfeeding: 500mcg

FOOD SOURCES:
Fortified cereal and bread, 1 slice or 1 cup: 100-670mcg
Beans and lentils, 1 cup: 260-360mcg
Spinach, cooked, ½ cup: 131mcg
Broccoli, cooked, 1 cup: 168mcg
Spaghetti, cooked, 1 cup: 167mcg
Orange juice, 1 cup: 75mcg

Vitamin C

FUNCTIONS:
→ Aids in maintenance of gums and
   healing of wounds
→ Helps make collagen
→ Enhances the absorption of iron
→ Antioxidant
→ Helps the immune system

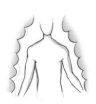

DAILY RECOMMENDATIONS:
All ages: 15-120mg
Teens: 65-75mg
Men: 90mg
Women: 75mg
Pregnant: 85mg
Breastfeeding: 120mg

FOOD SOURCES:
Yellow peppers, 1 cup: 283mg
Orange juice, 1 cup: 85-120mg
Cranberry juice cocktail, 1 cup: 107mg
Broccoli, cooked, 1 cup: 101mg
Strawberries, sliced, 1 cup: 106mg
Brussels sprouts, cooked, 1 cup: 97mg
Kiwi or orange, 1 medium: 70mg
Cantaloupe, 1 cup: 59mg
Mango, 1 medium: 57mg
Peas, cooked, 1 cup: 35mg
Raspberries and blackberries, 1 cup: 31mg
Soybeans, cooked, 1 cup: 31mg
Spinach, cooked, 1 cup: 31mg
Sweet potato, 1 medium: 29mg
Watermelon, 1 wedge: 23mg
Tomatoes, raw or canned, 1 cup: 23mg

Common Minerals (Calcium, Magnesium, Iron)

Calcium

FUNCTIONS:
➡ Helps build and maintain strong teeth and bones
➡ Can help slow bone loss due to aging
   (when combined with resistance training)
➡ Protects against osteoporosis
➡ Helps cell membrane stability
➡ Helps form blood clots in wounds
➡ Aids in weight loss and maintenance

DAILY RECOMMENDATIONS:
Children and teens: 1300mg
Adults: 1000mg
Older adults: 1200mg

FOOD SOURCES:
Milk, 1 cup: 285-300mg
Yogurt, 1 cup: 345mg
Calcium-fortified orange juice, 1 cup: 300mg
Rhubarb, cooked, 1/2 cup: 318mg
Enchilada, fast food, one serving: 324mg
Cheese, 1 ounce: 204mg
Macaroni and cheese, 1 cup: 300mg
Pudding, 1 cup: 300mg
Salmon, 3 ounces: 200mg
Sardines, 3 ounces: 200mg
Cottage Cheese, 1 cup: 150mg
Tofu, regular, 1/4 block: 163mg
Almonds, 1 ounce: 70mg
Baked beans, 1/2 cup: 64mg
Orange, 1 medium: 52mg
Cooked greens, 1/2 cup: 100mg

Magnesium

FUNCTIONS:
➡ Stabilize cellular structures
➡ Aids in metabolism of foods at the cellular level
➡ Aids in the synthesis of fatty acids and proteins
➡ Helps body get energy from ATP
➡ Aids in neuromuscular transmissions and activity
➡ Aids in muscle contraction

DAILY RECOMMENDATIONS:
Teens: 240-410mg
Adults: 310-400mg
Pregnant: 310-400mg

FOOD SOURCES:
Halibut, 1/2 fillet: 170mg
Spinach, cooked, 1 cup: 163mg
Oat bran muffin, 1 medium: 90mg
Brown rice, cooked, 1 cup: 84mg
Refried beans, 1 cup: 83mg
Orange juice, 6 ounces: 72mg
Baked potato, with skin, 1 medium: 57mg
Raisins, 1 cup: 46mg
Tofu, ¼ block: 30mg
Milk, 1 cup: 27mg
Fruits: 10-25mg

Magnesium is abundant in many foods, making deficiency in the United States unlikely.

Iron

FUNCTIONS:
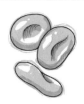
→ Makes hemoglobin for cells
→ Involved in all aspects of life
→ Aids in blood transport of oxygen
   and carbon dioxide

DAILY RECOMMENDATIONS:
Teenage girls: 15mg
Teenage boys: 11mg
Women: 18mg
Men: 8mg
Pregnant: 27mg
Breastfeeding: 9mg

FOOD SOURCES:
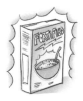
Fortified cereal, 1 serving: 1-22mg
Canned Clams, 3 ounces: 23mg
Beef tenderloin, 3 ounces: 3mg
Cooked soybeans, 1 cup: 8.8mg
Enriched rice, 1 cup: 9.7mg
Baked beans, 1 cup: 8.2mg
Enriched bagel, 1 whole: 5.4mg
Beans and lentils, 1 cup: 5-6.6mg
Blueberries, frozen, 1/2 cup: 4.5mg
Beef, ground, 3 ounces: 1.8mg
Spinach, cooked, 1/2 cup: 3.2mg
Chicken Breast, cooked, 3 ounces: 1.1mg
Turkey, cooked, 3 ounces: light 1.2mg, dark 2mg

Appendix E: Basal Metabolic Rate

Adapted from reference 23 and the American Dietetic Association's website
www.adaevidencelibrary.com/topic.cfm?cat=3209

Basal Metabolic Rate Calculations:

There are many different theories for calculating metabolic rate. Listed below are two of those options: (Also check askthedietitian.com for Healthy Body Calculator® estimate.)

HARRIS BENEDICT METHOD

➡ **Step 1: Calculate your basal metabolic rate (BMR).**

Women:
655 + (4.3 x weight in pounds) + (4.7 x height in inches) - (4.7 x age in years) = BMR

Men:
66 + (6.3 x weight in pounds) + (12.9 x height in inches) - (6.8 x age in years) = BMR

➡ **Step 2: Multiply your BMR by the following numbers, based on your activity level.**

Sedentary (little to no exercise): BMR x 1.2

Lightly active (light exercise or sports 1-3 days a week): BMR x 1.3

Moderately active (moderate exercise or sports 3-5 days a week): BMR x 1.4-1.5

Very active (intense work or exercise on a daily basis or for prolonged period): BMR x 1.5-1.7

Extra active (hard labor or athletic training): BMR x 1.7-1.8

➡ **Step 3: Add the numbers from Step 1 and Step 2 to figure out your daily calorie needs.**

OWEN'S METHOD

➡ **Men:** BMR = 879 + (10.2 x weight)

➡ **Women:** BMR = 795 + (7.18 x weight)

Appendix F: Calorie Dollars

To print this money, go to all-diets-work.com

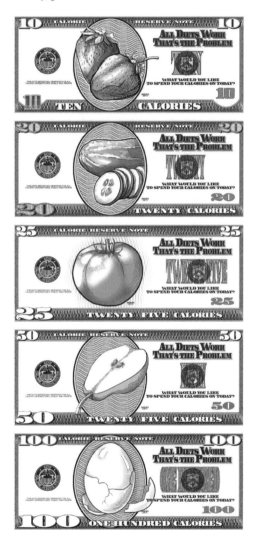

Appendix G: Food Diary Example

Food Journal

Date _____ Target Calories _____

Time	Food	Amount	Calories	Fat	Carbs	Protein
	Total:					

Exercise	
Type	**Time**

Water Intake (check one box per cup of water):

❏ ❏ ❏ ❏ ❏ ❏ ❏ ❏

Appendix H: Food Group Checklists

These food-group checklists can help you track how many servings from each food group you eat every day, so you can make sure your diet is healthy and balanced. The checklists are customized with target serving amounts for different levels of caloric intake. As you eat a food from the listed group, just place a check mark in one of the boxes. Then you can see at a glance how much you have eaten from each group and how many servings you still have left.

One note: these particular lists were made specifically to help people with diabetes keep blood sugar at a constant level, so the groups are separated based on their carbohydrate content. You will find some vegetables actually fall under the starch group instead of the vegetable group when counting for diabetes. If you have diabetes, you can find guidelines for categorizing foods on the Mayo Clinic Web site.* If diabetes is not an issue, simply count all vegetables in the vegetable group.

To print these charts, go to all-diets-work.com

*For a list of foods in each group, go to:
  http://www.mayoclinic.com/health/diabetes-diet/DA00069

Food Exchange Check List 1800 CALORIES

SUNDAY						
Starch / Carbohydrate (grain)						
Milk				▓	▓	▓
Fruit						
Meat						
Vegetable						▓
Fat					▓	▓
Free						

MONDAY						
Starch / Carbohydrate (grain)						
Milk				▓	▓	▓
Fruit						
Meat						
Vegetable						▓
Fat					▓	▓
Free						

TUESDAY						
Starch / Carbohydrate (grain)						
Milk				▓	▓	▓
Fruit						
Meat						
Vegetable						▓
Fat					▓	▓
Free						

WEDNESDAY						
Starch / Carbohydrate (grain)						
Milk				▓	▓	▓
Fruit						
Meat						
Vegetable						▓
Fat					▓	▓
Free						

Food Exchange Check List 1800 CALORIES CONT.

THURSDAY						
Starch / Carbohydrate (grain)						
Milk				■	■	■
Fruit						
Meat						
Vegetable						■
Fat					■	■
Free						

FRIDAY						
Starch / Carbohydrate (grain)						
Milk				■	■	■
Fruit						
Meat						
Vegetable						■
Fat					■	■
Free						

SATURDAY						
Starch / Carbohydrate (grain)						
Milk				■	■	■
Fruit						
Meat						
Vegetable						■
Fat					■	■
Free						

Food Exchange Check List 1500 CALORIES

SUNDAY						
Starch / Carbohydrate (grain)						
Milk				▓	▓	
Fruit				▓	▓	
Meat						
Vegetable					▓	▓
Fat					▓	▓
Free						

MONDAY						
Starch / Carbohydrate (grain)						
Milk				▓	▓	▓
Fruit				▓	▓	▓
Meat						
Vegetable					▓	▓
Fat					▓	▓
Free						

TUESDAY						
Starch / Carbohydrate (grain)						
Milk				▓	▓	▓
Fruit				▓	▓	▓
Meat						
Vegetable					▓	▓
Fat					▓	▓
Free						

WEDNESDAY						
Starch / Carbohydrate (grain)						
Milk				▓	▓	▓
Fruit				▓	▓	▓
Meat						
Vegetable					▓	▓
Fat					▓	▓
Free						

Food Exchange Check List 1500 CALORIES CONT.

THURSDAY						
Starch / Carbohydrate (grain)						
Milk						
Fruit						
Meat						
Vegetable						
Fat						
Free						

FRIDAY						
Starch / Carbohydrate (grain)						
Milk						
Fruit						
Meat						
Vegetable						
Fat						
Free						

SATURDAY						
Starch / Carbohydrate (grain)						
Milk						
Fruit						
Meat						
Vegetable						
Fat						
Free						

Food Exchange Check List 1200 CALORIES

SUNDAY						
Starch / Carbohydrate (grain)						
Milk				■	■	
Fruit					■	
Meat					□	■
Vegetable					■	
Fat				■	■	
Free						

MONDAY						
Starch / Carbohydrate (grain)						
Milk				■	■	
Fruit					■	
Meat					□	■
Vegetable					■	
Fat				■	■	
Free						

TUESDAY						
Starch / Carbohydrate (grain)						
Milk				■	■	
Fruit				□	■	
Meat					□	■
Vegetable					■	
Fat				■	■	
Free						

WEDNESDAY						
Starch / Carbohydrate (grain)						
Milk				■	■	
Fruit				□	■	
Meat					□	■
Vegetable					■	
Fat				■	■	
Free						

Food Exchange Check List 1200 CALORIES CONT.

THURSDAY						
Starch / Carbohydrate (grain)						
Milk						
Fruit						
Meat						
Vegetable						
Fat						
Free						

FRIDAY						
Starch / Carbohydrate (grain)						
Milk						
Fruit						
Meat						
Vegetable						
Fat						
Free						

SATURDAY						
Starch / Carbohydrate (grain)						
Milk						
Fruit						
Meat						
Vegetable						
Fat						
Free						

Appendix I: Stop Sign

To print this sign, go to all-diets-work.com

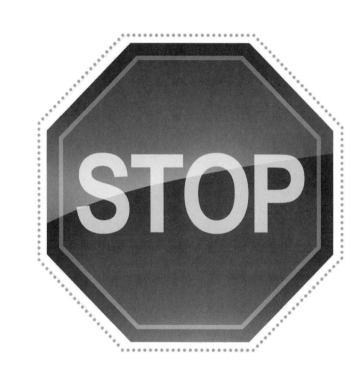

BLUEBERRY MUFFINS

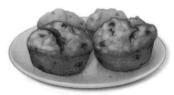

Yield: 12 muffins

1 cup oats
1½ cups flour (can use whole wheat)
½ cup brown sugar
2 teaspoons baking powder
½ teaspoon baking soda
½ teaspoon salt
1 egg
1 cup plus 2 tablespoons low-fat buttermilk
3 tablespoons oil
1 teaspoon vanilla
2 cups blueberries
½ cup sugar

1. Preheat oven to 400° and grease muffin tins.
2. Place oats in blender and blend until finely ground.
3. In large bowl, combine oats, flour, brown sugar, baking powder, baking soda, and salt. In small bowl, with fork, blend egg, buttermilk, oil, and vanilla; stir into flour mixture until flour is moistened. Fold in berries.
4. Spoon batter into muffin pan. Sprinkle with granulated sugar.
5. Bake 18 to 23 minutes until toothpick comes out clean. Invert onto wire rack.

Nutrition Information:
Serving Size: 1 muffin
Calories: 198
Total Fat: 4.6g
Saturated Fat: .8 gm
Cholesterol: 16 mg
Sodium: 181 mg
Carbohydrate 36 g
Fiber: 2 g
Protein: 4 g

CINNABEAN MUFFINS

(Don't worry, they'll never know!)
Yield: 18 muffins

1 cup sugar
2 tablespoons oil
½ cup applesauce
3 egg whites
1 egg
1 teaspoon vanilla
1 can pinto beans (pureed to
  pudding consistency)
2 cups flour
1½ tablespoon cinnamon
½ teaspoon baking powder
½ teaspoon baking soda
½ teaspoon salt
raisins (optional)

1. Preheat oven to 350° and
   grease muffin tins.
2. Mix sugar, oil, applesauce, eggs,
   egg whites, beans, and vanilla
   until smooth.
3. Add dry ingredients and stir just
   until blended. Add raisins if you're
   using them.
4. Bake 18 to 20 minutes, until
   toothpick comes out clean.
   Invert onto wire rack.

Nutrition Information:
Serving Size: 1 muffin
Calories: 208
Total Fat: 2.1 g
Saturated fat: .3 g
Cholesterol: 0 mg
Sodium: 119 mg
Carbohydrate: 40.2g
Fiber: 4.6g
Protein: 6.2g

WHOLE WHEAT PANCAKES

Yield: 14 pancakes
(compact disk size)

1 cup whole wheat kernels
1 cup milk
1 egg
¼ cup oil (or ¼ cup applesauce)
2 teaspoons sugar
1 teaspoon salt
3 teaspoons baking powder

1. Blend whole wheat and milk in
   blender on high speed for 3 minutes. Add another ½ cup milk,
   and blend 1 to 2 more minutes.
2. Add remaining ingredients and
   blend until smooth.
3. Pour on hot greased griddle
   and cook until golden brown
   on both sides.

Nutrition Information:
Serving Size: 1 large pancake or
  2 small pancakes
Calories: 43
Total Fat: 1.5g
Saturated Fat: .3g
Cholesterol: 14 mg
Sodium: 184 mg
Carbohydrate: 7g
Fiber: 1.8g
Protein: 2g

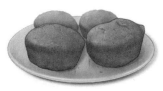

BUTTERSCOTCH
OATMEAL COOKIES

Yield: 36 cookies

¾ cup applesauce
¾ cup packed brown sugar
½-¾ cup white sugar
1 egg (or 2 egg whites)
1 teaspoon vanilla
1 ½ cups flour
1 teaspoon baking soda
1 teaspoon salt
2 teaspoons cinnamon
¼ teaspoon nutmeg (optional)
3 cups quick oats
1 package butterscotch chips

1. Preheat oven to 350°.
2. Beat applesauce and sugars until
   well blended. Beat in egg and vanilla.
3. Add dry ingredients, mix well. Fold
   in butterscotch chips.
4. Drop by rounded spoonfuls onto
   greased cookie sheets. Bake 8
   to10 minutes.

Nutrition Information:
Serving Size: 1 cookie
Calories: 111
Total Fat: .9g
Saturated Fat: .3g
Cholesterol: 6 mg
Sodium: 139 mg
Total Carbohydrate: 24g
Fiber: 1g
Protein: 1.6g

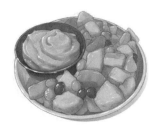

FRUIT DIP

Yield: 4 cups

1 package (8-ounce) fat-free cream
cheese, softened
2 to 7 ounces marshmallow ice cream
topping (can use marshmallow fluff,
and beat longer to make it smooth)
1 cup fat-free strawberry yogurt
1 tub (8 ounce) fat-free Cool Whip

1. Whip cream cheese until light
   and fluffy.
2. Add marshmallow topping and
   cool whip and mix until well-
   blended.
3. Add Cool Whip and mix until
   smooth. Refrigerate until ready
   to serve.

Nutrition Information:
Serving Size: 2 rounded tablespoons
Calories: 29
Total Fat: 0g
Sodium: 61 mg
Total Carbohydrate: 5.4g
Fiber: 0 g
Protein: 1.3g

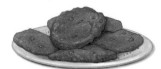

CHIP DIP

Yield: 3 cups

1 can beans (pinto is great,
  but any kind work)
1 cup salsa
¾ cup grated cheese

1. Mix all together in a blender
   until relatively smooth. Heat until
   cheese melts.
2. Serve warm or cold with chips.

Nutrition Information:
Serving Size: 1 1/2 tablespoons
Calories: 28
Total Fat: 1g
Saturated fat: .6g
Cholesterol: 3 mg
Sodium: 89 mg
Total Carbohydrate: 3.2g
Fiber: 1g
Protein: 1.7g

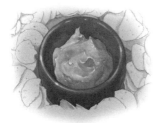

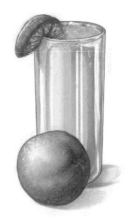

DREAMSICLE SMOOTHIE

Yield: 5 cups

2 cups frozen oranges (yes, you can
  freeze peeled oranges in sections)
2 cups skim milk (add more or less
  for desired consistency)
½ cup lowfat vanilla yogurt
½ cup sugar (or other sweetener
  of your choice)

Place all together in blender and
blend until smooth

Nutrition Information:
Serving Size: 1 cup
Calories: 125
Total Fat: .2g
Saturated Fat: .1g
Cholesterol: 3 mg
Sodium: 61 mg
Total Carbohydrate: 26.7g
Fiber: 1.7 g
Protein: 5.5 g

STRAWBERRY BANANA SMOOTHIE

Yield: 5 cups

2 cups frozen strawberries
2 cups skim milk
1 frozen banana
1 teaspoon vanilla
¼ cup sugar
1 small container (6 ounce)
   strawberry yogurt

Place all ingredients in blender and blend until smooth.

Nutrition Information:
Serving Size: 1 cup
Calories: 132
Total Fat: .3g
Saturated Fat: .1g
Cholesterol: 3 mg
Sodium: 59 mg
Total Carbohydrate: 28.8g
Fiber: 1.8g
Protein: 5g

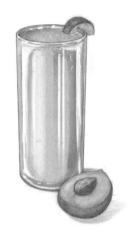

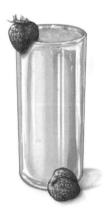

PEACHY KEEN SMOOTHIE

Yield: 5 cups

2 cups frozen, sliced peaches
2 cups milk
1 frozen banana
1/2 cup sugar
1 teaspoon vanilla

Place all ingredients in blender and blend until smooth.

Nutrition Information:
Serving Size: 1 cup
Calories: 162
Total Fat: .5g
Saturated Fat: .2g
Cholesterol: 2 mg
Sodium: 52 mg
Total Carbohydrates: 37g
Fiber: 1.6g
Protein: 4.4g

Appendix K: Meal-Planning Worksheet

Day/Dinner Menu	Recipe Source	Groceries Needed
MONDAY		
TUESDAY		
WEDNESDAY		
THURSDAY		
FRIDAY		
SATURDAY		
SUNDAY		

References

Section 1: The Diet Dilemma

1. *BRFSS - CDC's Behavioral Risk Factor Surveillance System.* CDC, 16 May 2011. Web. 29 May 2011. <http://www.cdc. gov/brfss/>.

2. Mokdad, AH, et al. " The spread of the obesity epidemic in the United States." *JAMA* 282.10 (1999): 1519-22.

3. Mokdad AH, et al. "The continuing epidemics of obesity and diabetes in the United States." *JAMA*. 286.10 (2001): 1519–22.

4. Mokdad AH, et al. "Prevalence of obesity, diabetes, and obesity-related health risk factors." *JAMA*: 289.1 (2003): 76–79.

5. CDC. "State-Specific Prevalence of Obesity Among Adults— United States, 2005." *MMWR* 55.36 (2006): 985–988.

6. Gupta, Sanjay, and Elizabeth Cohen. "CDC: More People Obese Now than in 2007." *The Chart.* CNN, 4 Aug. 2010. Web. 29 May 2011. <http://thechart.blogs.cnn.com/2010/08/04/ cdc-more-people-obese-now-than-in-2007>.

7. Malnick, SDH, H. Knobler. "The Medical Complications of Obesity." QJM 2006 99(9):565-579.

8. "Latest Increase in US Obesity Rate Will Mean More

Cancers, Experts Warn." *ICR Annual Research Conference.* American Institute for Cancer Research, 4 Aug. 2010. Web. 29 May 2011. Path: aicr.org;Press; Press Releases.

9. Gortmaker, SL, A Must, JM Perrin, AM Sobol, and WH Dietz. "Social and economic consequences of overweight in adolescence and young adulthood." *New England Journal of Medicine* 329(14) Sept. (1993): 1008–1012

10. Definition of *diet* at YourDictionary.com. LoveToKnow Corp., n.d. Web. 29 May 2011. <yourdictionary.com/diet>.

11. Sacks, FM, GA Bray, VJ Carey, SR Smith, and DH Ryan, et al. "Comparison of weight-loss diets with different compositions of fat, protein, and carbohydrates." *New England Journal of Medicine* 360.9 26 Feb. (2009): 859-73.

12. Mann, T, AJ Tomiyama, E Westling, AM Lew, B Samuels, and J Chatman. "Medicare's Search for Effective Obesity Treatments: Diets Are Not the Answer." *American Psychology* 62.3 Apr. (2007): 220-33.

13. Rolland-Cachera, MF, H Thibault, JC Souberbielle, D Soulie, et al. "Massive obesity in adolescents: Dietary interventions and behaviors associated with weight regain at 2 y follow-up." *Int J Obes Relat Metab Disord.* 28.4 Apr (2004): 514-9.

14. Saelens, B, J Sallis, D Wilfley, K Patrick, J Cella, and R Buchta. "Behavioral weight control for overweight adolescents initiated in primary care." *Obesity Research* 10 (2002): 22-32.

15. Olson, M.B. et al. "Weight cycling and high-density lipoprotein cholesterol in women: Evidence of an adverse effect." *Journal of the American College of Cardiology* 36.5 Nov. (2002): 1565-1571.

Section 2: Principles of Weight Management

16. Grave, R, S Calugi, A Ruocco, and G Marchesini. "Night eating syndrome and weight loss outcome in obese patients." *Int J Eat Disord*. Feb (2010). Epub.

17. Striegel-Moore, RH, DL Franko, D Thompson, S Affenito, A May, and HC Kraemer. "Exploring the typology of night eating syndrome." *Int J Eat Disord*. 41.5 July (2008): 411-8.

18. Boutelle, K, D Neumark-Sztainer, M Story, and M Resnick. "Weight control behaviors among obese, overweight, and non overweight adolescents." *J Pediatr Psychol*. 27.6 Sep. (2002): 531-40.

19. Silva, MN, D Markland, EV Carraca, PN Viera, SR Coutinho, et al. "Exercise Autonomous motivation predicts three-year weight loss in women." *Med Sci Sports Exerc*. Aug 2 (2010). Epub.

20. De Castro, JM. "The time of day of food intake influences overall intake in humans." *J Nutr*. 134.1 Jan (2004): 104-11.

21. USDA.gov. USDA. Web. 29 May 2011. <http://www.mypyramid.gov/pyramid/grains_amount.aspx>.

22. *Dietary Reference Intakes for Energy, Carbohydrate, Fiber, Fat, Fatty Acids, Cholesterol, Protein, and Amino Acids (Macronutrients)*. Food and Nutrition Board, 2005, p 265. Available from<http://www.nap.edu/openbook.php?record_id=10490&page=265>.

23. Mahan, LK. *Krause's food and nutrition therapy*. 12th ed. St. Louis: Saunders, 2009. Print.

24. American Dietetic Association. "Health implications of dietary fiber—position of ADA." *Journal of the American Dietetic Association*. Oct. 2008: 1716-1731. Available from <http://www.eatright.com>.

REFERENCES

25. Institute of Medicine, Food and Nutrition Board. *Dietary reference intakes for energy, carbohydrates, fiber, fat, protein, and amino acids (macronutrient).* Washington, DC: National Academies Press, 2002.

26. eatright.org. American Dietetic Association, n.d. Web. 29 May 2011. <http://www.eatright.org/>

27. Bauer, LR, and J Waldrop. "Trans fat intake in children: risks and recommendations." *Pediatr Nurs.* 35.6 Nov-Dec (2009):346-51

28. Remig, V, B Ranklin B, S Margolis, G Kostas, T Nece, and JC Street. "Trans fats in America: a review of their use, consumption, health implications, and regulation." *J Am Diet Assoc.* 110.4 Apr. (2010): 585-92.

29. Ammerman, A, et al. "Counseling to promote a healthy diet [Internet]." Rockville (MD): Agency for healthcare Research and Quality (US); 2002 Apr.

30. Theorell-Haglow, J, C Berne, C Janson, C Sahlin, and E Lindberg. "Associations between short sleep duration and central obesity in women." *Sleep.* 33.5 May (2010): 593-8.

31. Anic, GM, L Titus-Ernstoff, PA Newcomb, A Trentham-Dietz, and KM Egan. "Sleep duration and obesity in a population-based study." *Sleep Med.* 11.5 May (2010:447-51.

32. Hairston, KG, et al. "Sleep duration and five-year abdominal fat accumulation in a minority cohort: the IRAS family study." *Sleep.* 33.3 Mar. (2010):289-95.

33. Tian, Z, et al. "Sleep duration and hyperglycemia among obese and nonobese children aged 3 to 6 years." *Arch Pediatr Adolesc Med.* 164.1 Jan. (2010):46-52.

34. Phillips, BG, M Kato, K Narkiewicz, I Choe, and VK Somers.

"Increases in leptin levels, sympathetic drive, and weight gain in obstructive sleep apnea." *Am J Physiol Heart Circ Physiol.* 279.1 Jul.(2000): H234-7.

35. Levy P, MR Bonsignore, and J Eckel. "Sleep, sleep-disordered breathing and metabolic consequences." *Eur Respir J.* 34.5 Nov (2009):1209-10.

36. Chen, MY, EK Wang, and YJ Jeng. "Adequate sleep among adolescents is positively associated with health status and health-related behaviors." *Chang Gung Institute of Technology.* Kwei-Shan, Taoyuan, Taiwan.

37. Van Cauter R, and KL Knutson. "Sleep and the epidemic of obesity in children and adults. Eur J Endocrinol." Dec. (2008) 159 Suppl 1:S59-66.

38. Schmid SM, Hallschmid M, Jauch-Chara K, Born J, Schultes B. "A single night of sleep deprivation increases ghrelin levels and feelings of hunger in normal-weight healthy men." *J Sleep Res.* 2008 Sep;17(3):331-4.

39. Bosy-Westphal A, Hinrichs, S, Jauch-Chara K, Hitze B, Later W, Wilms B, Settler U, Peters A, Kiosz D, Muller MJ. "Influence of partial sleep deprivation on energy balance and insulin sensitivity in healthy women." *Obes Facts.* 2008;1(5):266-73.

40. Spiegel K, Tasali E, Penev P, Van Cauter E. "Sleep curtailment in healthy young men is associated with decreased leptin levels, elevated ghrelin levels, and increased hunger and appetite." *Ann Intern Med.* 2004 Dec 7;141(11):846-50.

41. Nishiura C, Noguchi J, Hashimoto H. "Dietary patterns only partially explain the effect of short sleep duration on the incidence of obesity." *Sleep.* 2010 Jun 1;33(6):753-7.

42. Dzaja A, Dalal MA, Himmerich H, Uhr M, Pollmacher T,

Schuld A. "Sleep enhances nocturnal plasma ghrelin levels in healthy subjects." *Am J Physiol EndocrinolMetab.* 2004 Jun;286(6):E963-7.

43. Motivala SJ, Tomiyama AJ, Ziegler M, Khandrika S, Irwin MR. "Nocturnal levels of ghrelin and leptin and sleep in chronic insomnia." *Psychoneuroendocrinology.* 2009 May;34(4):540-5.

44. Mann, Denise. "Sleep and Weight Gain." *WebMD.* WebMD, 2009. Web. 29 May 2011. <http://www. webmd.com/sleep-disorders/excessive-sleepiness-10/ lack-of-sleep-weight-gain>.

45. Mayo Clinic Staff. " Exercise for weight loss: Calories burned in 1 hour" *Mayo Clinic: Weight Loss.* Mayo Foundation for Medical Education and Research, 1 December 2009. Web. 29 May 2011. < http://www.mayoclinic.com/health/exercise/ SM00109>.

46. O'Donovan G, Blazevich AJ, Boreham C, Cooper AR, Crank H, Ekelund U, Fox KR, Gately P, Giles-Corti B, Gill JM, Hamer M, McDermott I, Murphy M, Mutrie N, Reilly JJ, Saxtion JM, Stamatakis E. "The abc of physical activity for health: a consensus statement from the British Association of Sport and Exercise Sciences." *J Sports Sci.* 2010 Apr;28(6):573-91.

47. Rees DI, Sabia JJ. "Exercise and adolescent mental health: new evidence from longitudinal data." *J Ment Health Policy Econ.* 2010 Mar;13(1):13-25.

48. Akkary, E, Cramer T, Chaar O, Raiput K, Yu S, Dziura J, Roberts K, Duffy A, Bel R. "Survey of the effective exercise habits of the formerly obese." *JSLS.* 2010 Jan-Mar;14(1):106-14. Epub 2010 Apr 21.

49. Blake H, Mo P, Malik S, Thomas S. "How effective are physical activity interventions for alleviating depressive symptoms in older people? A systematic review." *Clin Rehabil.* 2009 Oct;23(10):873-87.

50. Tudor-Locke C, Lutes L. "Why do pedometers work?: a reflection upon the factors related to successfully increasing physical activity." *Sports Med.* 2009;39(12):981-93.

51. Mayo Clinic Staff. "Exercise: 7 benefits of regular physical activity." *Mayo Clinic: Fitness.* Mayo Foundation for Medical Education and Research, 5 July 2009. Web. 29 May 2011. <http://www.mayoclinic.com/health/exercise/HQ01676>.

52. Doyle, J. Andrew. "The Benefits of Exercise." *The Exercise and Physical Fitness Page.* Georgia State University, 6 Nov. 1997. Web. 29 May 2011. <http://www2.gsu.edu/~wwwfit/benefits.html>.

53. Wilbert, Caroline. "Exercise vs. Diets: Weighing the Benefit." Healthy Aging Health Center. *WebMD*, 19 Sept. 2008. Web. 29 May 2011. <http://www.webmd.com/healthy-aging/news/20080918/exercise-vs-dietsweighing-the-benefits>.

54. Hendrick, Bill. "Even a Little Exercise Fights Obesity." Health and Fitness. *WebMD*, 6 Nov. 2009. Web. 29 May 2011. <http://www.webmd.com/fitness-exercise/news/20091106/even-a-little-exercise-fights-obesity>.

55. O'Donoghue K JM, Fournier PA, Guelfi KJ. "Lack of effecgt of exercise time of day on acute energy intake in healthy men." *Int J Sport Nutr Exerc Metab.* 2010 Aug; 20(4):350-6

56. Ciccolo JT, Pettee Gabriel KK, Macera C, Ainsworth BE. "Association between self-reported resistance training and self-rated health in a national sample of U.S. men and women." *J Phys Act Health* 2010 May:7(3):289-98.

REFERENCES

57. Akkary E, Cramer T, Chaar O, Rajput K, Yu S, Dziura J, Roberts K, Duggy A, Bell R. "Survery of the effective exercise habits of the formerly obese." *JSLS*. 2010 Jan-Mar;14(1):106-14. Epub 2010 Apr 21.

58. Walker KZ, O'Dea K, Gomez M, Girgis S, Colagiuri R. "Diet and exercise in the prevention of diabetes." *J Hum Nutr Die*. 2010 Aug;23(4):344-52. Epub 2010 Mar 23.

59. Rigamonti AE, Agosti R, De Col A, Marazzi N, Lafortuna CL, Cella SG, Muller EE, Sartorio A. "Changes in plasma levels of ghrelin, leptin and other hormonal and metabolic paramerters following standardized breakfast, lunch and physical exercise before and after a multidisciplinary weight-reduction intervention in obese adolescents." *J Endocrinol Invest*. 2010 Mar 25. Epub.

60. King NA, Caudwell PP, Hopkins M, Stubbs JR, Naslund E, Blundell JE. "Dual-process action of exercise on appetite control: increase in orexigenic drive but improvement in meal0induced satiety." *Am J Clin Nutr*. 2009 Oct;90(4):921-7. Epub.

61. Wing RR, Phelan S. "Long-term weight loss maintenance." *Am J Clin Nutr*. 2005 Jul;82(1 Suppl):222S-225S.

62. Schmidt D, Biwer C, Kalscheuer L. "Effects of long versus short bout exercise of fitness and weight loss in overweight females." *J Am Col Nut*. 2001; 20(5): 494-501.

63. Banquet G, Gamelin FX, Mucci P, Thevenet D, Van Praach E, Berthoin S. "Continuous vs. interval aerobic training in 8- to 11-year-old children." *J Strength Cond Res*. 2010 May;24(5):1381-8.

REFERENCES

Section 3: Tools

64. Neuhouser ML, Tinker L, Shaw PA, Schoeller D, Bingham SA, Horn LV, Beresford SA, Caan B, Thomson C, Satterfield S, Kuller L, Heiss G, Smit E, Sarto G, Ockene J, Stefanick ML, Assaf A, Runswick S, Prentice RL. "Use of recovery biomarkers to calibrate nutrient consumption self-reports in the Women's Health Initiative." *Am J Epidemiol.* 2008 May 15;167(10):1247-59. Epub.

65. Vereecken C, Dohogne S, Covents M, Maes L. "How accurate are adolescents in portion-size estimation using the computer tool Young Adolescents' Nutrition Assessment on Computer (YANA-C)?" *Br J Nutr.* 2010 Jun;103(12):1844-50.

66. Wansink B, Painter JE, North J. "Bottomless bowls: why visual cues of portion size may influence intake." *Obes Res.* 2005 Jan;13(1):93-100.

67. Japur CC, Diez-Garcia RW. "Food energy content influences food portion size estimation by nutrition students." *J Hum Nutr Diet.* 2010 Jun;23(3):272-6.

68. Johnson RK, Friedman AB, Harvey-Berino J, Gold BC, McKenzie D. "Participation in a behavioral weight-loss program worsens the prevalence and severity of underreporting among obese and overweight women." *J Am Diet Assoc.* 2005 Dec;105(12)1948-51.

69. Bedard D, Shatenstein B, Nadon S. "Underreporting of energy intake from a self-administered food-frequency questionnaire completed by adults in Montreal." *Public Health Nutr.* 2004 Aug;7(5):675-81.

70. Harnack L, Steffen L, Arnett DK, Gao S, Luepker RV. "Accuracy of estimation of large food portions." *J Am Diet Assoc.* 2004 May;104(5):804-6.

REFERENCES

71. Mendez MA, Wynter S, Wilks R, Forrester T. "Under-and overreporting of energy is related to obesity, lifestyle factors and food group intakes in Jamaican adults." *Public Health Nutr.* 2004 Feb;7(1):9-19.

72. Scagliusi RB, Polacow VO, Artioli GG, Benatti FB, Lancha AH Jr. "Selective underreporting of energy intake in women: magnitude, determinants, and effect of training." *J Am Diet Assoc.* 2003 Oct;103(10):1306-13

73. Lissner L. "Measuring food intake in studies of obesity." *Public Health Nutr.* 2002 Dec;5(6A):889-92.

74. Champagne CM, Bray GA, Kurtz AA, Monteiro JB, Tucker E, Volaufovs J, Delany JP. "Energy intake and energy expenditure: a controlled study comparing dietitians and non-dietitians." *J Am Diet Assoc.* 2002 Oct;102(10):1428–32.

75. Kant AK. "Nature of dietary reporting by adults in the third National Health and Nutrition Examination Survey, 1988–1994." *J Am Coll Nutr.* 2002 Aug;21(4):315-27.

76. Rzewnicki R, Vanden Auweele Y, De Bourdeaudhuij I. "Addressing overreporting on the International Physical Activity Questionnaire (IPAQ) telephone survey with a population sample." *Public Health Nutr.* 2003 May;6(3):299-305.

77. McMurray RG, Ward DS, Elder JP, Lytle LA, Strikmiller PK, Baggett CD, Young DR. "Do overweight girls over-report physical activity?" *Am J Health Behav.* 2008 Sep-Oct;32(5):538-46.

78. Bleich SN, Huizinga MM, Beach MC, Cooper LA"Patient use of weight-management activities: a comparison of patient and physician assessments." *Patient Educ Couns.* 2010 Jun;79(3):344-50. Epub.

79. Bogl LH, Pietiläinen KH, Rissanen A, Kaprio J. "Improving

the accuracy of self-reports on diet and physical exercise: the co-twin control method." *Twin Res Hum Genet.* 2009 Dec;12(6):531-40.

80. Nielson SJ, Popkin BM. "Patterns and trends in foods portion sizes, 1977-1998." *JAM.* 2003;289(4):450-453.

81. Young LR, Nestle M. "The contribution of expanding portion sizes to the US Obesity Epidemic." *Am J Public Health.* 2002 Feb;92(2):246-249.

82. Steenhuis IH, Vermeer WM. "Portion size: review and framework for interventions." *Int J Behav Nutr Phys Act.* 2009 Aug 21;6:58.

83. Schwartz J, Byrd-Bredbenner C. "Portion distortion: typical portion sizes selected by young adults." *J Am Diet Assoc.* 2006 Sep;106(9):1412-8.

84. Clark A, Franklin J, Pratt I, McGrice M. "Overweight and obesity - use of portion control in management." *Aust Fam Physician* 2010 June(39)6:401-11.

85. Kazaks A, Stern JS. "Obesity: food intake." *Prim Care.* 2003 Jun;30(2):301-16, vi.

86. Hannum SM, Carson LA, Evans EM, Canene KA, Petr EL, Bui L, Erdman JW. "Use of portion-controlled entrees enhances weight loss in women." *Obes Res* 2004; 12; 538-546

87. Levitsky DA, Youn T. "The more food young adults are served, the more they overeat." *J Nutr* 2004; 134: 2546-2549.

88. Rolls BJ, Morris EL, Roe LS. "Portion size of food affects energy intake in normal-weight and overweight men and women." *Am J Clin Nutr* 2002; 76-1207-1213.

89. Rolls, B. *The volumetrics weight control plan.* New York: HarperCollins, 2000.

REFERENCES

90. Rolls, B. *The volumetrics weight control plan*. New York: HarperCollins, 2005.

91. U.S. Department of Health and Human Services and U.S. Department of Agriculture. *Dietary Guidelines for Americans, 2005*. 6th Edition, Washington, DC: U.S. Government Printing Office, January 2005.

92. Rolls BJ, Roe LS, Meengs JS. "Salad and satiety: energy density and portion size of a first course salad affect energy intake at lunch." *J Am Diet Assoc.* 2004 Oct;104(10):1570-6.

93. Flood-Obbagy JE, Rolls BJ. "The effect of fruit in different forms on energy intake and satiety at a meal." *Appetite.* 2009 Apr;52(2):416-22.

94. Flood JE, Rolls BJ. "Soup preloads in a variety of forms reduce meal energy intake." *Appetite.* 2007 Nov;49(3):626-34.

95. Foco, Z. *Water with Lemon*. Onsted:HNI, 2006.

96. Tate DF, Wing RR, Wiett RA. "Using Internet technology to deliver a behavioral weight loss program." *JAMA.* 2001;285:1172-1177.

97. Carels RA, Young KM, Coit C, Clayton AM, Spencer A, Hobbs M. "Can following the caloric restriction recommendations from the Dietary Guidelines for Americans help individuals lose weight?" *Eat Behav.* 2008;9:328-335.

98. Hollis JF, Gullion CM, Stevens VJ, Brantley PJ, Appel LJ, Ard JD, Champagne CM, Dalcin A, Erlinger TP, Funk K, Laferriere D, Lin PH, Loria CM, Samuel-Hodge C, Vollmer WM, Svetkey LP. "Weight loss during the intensive intervention phase of the weight –loss maintenance trial." *Am J Prev Med.* 2008;35:118-126.

99. Shay LE, Seibert D, Watts D, Sbrocco T, Pagliara C.

REFERENCES

"Adherence and weight loss outcomes associated with food-exercise diary preference in a military weight management program." *Eat Behav.* 2009;10:220-227.

100. Kaiser Permanente. "Keeping A Food Diary Doubles Diet Weight Loss, Study Suggests." *Science Daily.* Science Daily, 8 July 2008. Web. 29 May 2011. <http://www.sciencedaily.com/releases/2008/07/080708080738.htm>.

101. Cho S. Dietrich M, Brown CJP, Clark CA, Block G. "The effect of breakfast type on total daily energy intake and body mass index: Results from the Third National Health and Nutrition Examination Survey (NHANESIII)." *J Am Coll Nutr* 2003; 22(4) 296-302.

102. Ma Y, Bertone ER, Stanek EJ, Reed GW, Hebert JR, Cohen NL, Merriam PA, Ockene IS. "Association between eating patterns and obesity in a free-living US adult population." *Am J Epidemiol.* 2003; 158(1):85-92.

103. Schlundt DG, Hill JO, Sbrocco T, Pope-Cordle J, Sharp T. "The role of breakfast in the treatment of obesity: a random-ized clinical trial." *Am J Clin Nutr.* 1992; 55:645-651.

104. Sitzman K. "Eating breakfast helps sustain weight loss." *AAOHN J.* 2006 Mar; 54(3): 136.

105. Mattes RD. "Ready-to-eat cereal used as a meal replacement promotes weight loss in humans." *J Am Coll Nutr.* 2002 Dec;21(6):570-7

106. Ortega RM, Lopez-Sobaler AM, Andres P, Rodriguez-Rodrigues E, Aparicio A, Bermejo LM. "Increasing con-sumption of breakfast cereal improves thiamine status in overweight/obese women following a hypocaloric diet." *Int J Food Sci Nutr.* 2009;60(1):69-79.

107. Schlundt DG, Hill JO, Sbrocco T, Pope-Cordle J, Sharp T.

"The role of breakfast in the treatment of obesity: a randomized clinical trial." *Am J Clin Nutr.* 1992 Mar;55(3):645-51.

108. Woodruff SJ, Hanning RM, Lambraki I, Storey KE, McCargar L. "Healthy eating index-c is compromised among adolescents with body weight concerns, weight loss dieting, and meal skipping." *Body Image.* 2008 Dec;5(4): 404-8. Epub.

109. Wansink B, Painter JE, North J. "Bottomless bowls: why visual cues of portion size may influence intake." *Obes Res.* 2005 Jan;13(1): 93-100.

110. Ebrecht M, Hextall J, Kirtley LG, Taylor A, Dyson M, Weinman J. "Perceived stress and cortisol levels predict speed of wound healing in healthy male adults." *Psychoneuroendocrinology.* July 2004.

111. Mayo Clinic Staff. "Stress: Constant Stress Puts Your Health at Risk." *Mayo Clinic: Stress Management.* Mayo Foundation for Medical Education and Research, 26 Feb. 2009. Web. 29 May 2011. <http://www.mayoclinic.com/health/stress/SR00001>.

112. Covey, SR. *The Seven Habits of Highly Effective People.* New York: Simon and Schuster, 1989.

113. Frankl, V. *Man's Search for Meaning.* New York: Simon and Schuster, 1959.

114. Turner-McGrievy GM, Barnard ND, Scialli AR. "A two-year randomized weight loss trial comparing a vegan diet to a more moderate low-fat diet." *Obesity* (Silver Spring). 2007 Sep;15(9):2276-81.

115. Linde JA, Jeffery RW, French SA, Pronk NP, Boyle RG. "Self-weighing in weight gain prevention and weight loss trial." *Ann Behav Med.* 2005;30:210-216.

REFERENCES

116. Wing RR, Tate DF, Gorin AA, Raynor HA, Fava JL. "A self-regulation program for maintenance of weight loss." *N Engl J Med.* 2006;355:1563-1571.

117. Continuum Health Partners website. Bowel Function Dietary Fiber Chart. http://www.wehealny.org/healthinfo/dietaryfiber/fibercontentchart.html.

MY NOTES AND GOALS

_____

_____

_____

_____

_____

_____

_____

_____

_____

_____

_____

_____

_____

_____

_____

_____

_____

_____

_____

_____

_____

_____

_____

_____

_____

_____

_____

_____

_____

_____

_____

_____

_____

_____

_____

_____

_____

_____

_____

_____

_____

_____

MY NOTES AND GOALS

About the Author

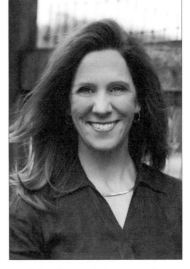

Jen Brewer is a registered dietician with over a decade of experience teaching about healthy eating.

She teaches in one-on-one counseling sessions and group seminars, and she has appeared on radio programs and in newspapers and magazines.

Her goal is to help people, young and old, gain personal motivation and finally see lasting results.

Visit WWW.ALL-DIETS-WORK.COM.